Management
in Nursing

A Vital Link in the
Health Care System

Management in Nursing

A Vital Link in the Health Care System

Carolyn Chambers Clark, R.N., Ed.D.

Formerly Graduate School of Nursing
Pace University

Carole A. Shea, R.N., M.S.

College of Nursing
Rutgers–The State University

McGraw-Hill Book Company

New York St. Louis San Francisco Auckland Bogotá Düsseldorf
Johannesburg London Madrid Mexico Montreal New Delhi
Panama Paris São Paulo Singapore Sydney Tokyo Toronto

MANAGEMENT IN NURSING:
A Vital Link in the Health Care System

234567890 DODO 7832109

Library of Congress Cataloging in Publication Data

Clark, Carolyn Chambers.
  Management in nursing.

  Includes index.
  1. Nursing service administration. I. Shea, Carole
A., joint author. II. Title.
RT89.C55   658'.91'61073   78-19098
ISBN 0-07-011135-9

This book was set in Times Roman by The Book Studio Inc. The editor was
Orville W. Haberman, Jr.; the cover was designed by Toni Goldmark; the production
supervisor was Jeanne Selzam.
R. R. Donnelley & Sons Company was printer and binder.

To Bill and John

Contents

PART 2
NURSING ALTERNATIVES WITHIN THE SYSTEM

List of Contributors

PAT ARCHBOLD, R.N., M.S., currently a doctoral student, has practiced community health nursing in free clinics, neighborhood health centers, and health screening projects.

CAROLYN CHAMBERS CLARK, R.N., Ed.D., teaches assertiveness, group dynamics, and systems concepts to nurses. She is author of numerous articles and five other books.

WILLIAM F. CLARK, M.B.A., M.S. (Finance) is president of his own company, and financial advisor to and director of several corporations.

RITA DE COTIIS, R.N., M.A., is the Executive Director of Nursing Service Inc. She is the current President of the Home Health Agency Assembly of New Jersey.

RUTH R. GREENBERG EDELSTEIN, R.N., Ph.D., is a research director and educator. Some of her many publications concern the development of grounded theory and the democratization of nursing research.

GUS W. GRAMMAS, Ph.D., teaches operations research, business policy, and strategic planning. His publications, research, and consultation concern management in urban systems and health services.

KATHY HARTNETT, R.N., M.S., is a clinical specialist in an acute psychiatric service based in a community mental health center. She has published and has given workshops in crisis intervention for nurses.

JOHN M. OAKES, B.S.F.S., is Division Executive in the International Department of a major bank. He uses performance contracting as a tool for developing junior officers.

VIRGINIA O'HALLORAN, R.N., M.S., teaches family health nursing and designs performance examinations for nurses. She is a member of the Hudson Valley Health Systems Agency.

MARIAN MARTIN PETTENGILL, R.N., M.S., is a teacher, clinical specialist, and consultant on mental health. She has served in official capacity for several state nursing associations.

JOAN K. SCHROEDER, R.N., M.A., is the Director of the Visiting Nurses of Northern Bergen County, Inc., New Jersey.

CAROLE A. SHEA, R.N., M.S., teaches family systems, nursing intervention, and management concepts. She presents seminars on the use of action research and the nurse's role in changing health organizations.

SHELLEY VAN KEMPEN, R.N., M.S., is a clinical specialist in oncology at a large hospital. She has developed the role of the nurse advocate in her practice and research.

Preface

Management in nursing is the process of linking together work groups that are organized around specific problems or issues related to nursing practice. Nurses cannot be effective managers by merely taking or being assigned the positions of head nurse, department head, administrator, or director of nursing. Effective management in complex health care systems requires that the nurse have knowledge and skills related to management functions, organization environments, communication and decision making, and mastery of a repertoire of roles to implement new alternatives and innovations of change. Lacking these, the nurse manager often resorts to avoidance or compliance behaviors which result in uncreative, reactive, illness-oriented nursing care.

Three types of change have dictated the need for this book: social changes, institutional changes, and administration changes in approaches to management. These changes include legislation encouraging greater consumer input in the health care decision-making process; an increased awareness among nurses of their professional responsibilities to direct and implement the changes suggested by health care legislation; the growth of independent nursing practice as exemplified by the establishment of peer relationships with other health professionals, the development of nurse practitioner programs, and updated nurse practice acts; the consumerism movement and greater attention to clients' rights; an emphasis on preventive and community-based health care; changed technology and the resultant ethical and human relations concerns; and a shift in the base of administration and management to small group theory and systems analysis.

Because of these changes, we have tried to present a systems theory framework within which we discuss the existing process of management as it pertains to health care systems, organizational environment, planning, leadership, and evaluation. A major portion of the book looks forward to try to delineate nursing alternatives within the system.

This book can be used as a basic text in baccalaureate programs for such introductory courses as nursing leadership, senior clinical nursing, health care delivery systems, nursing management, and nursing administration. It might also be useful for other baccalaureate courses dealing with leadership, environmental management, or personnel management.

At the graduate level the book could be used as a basic text in courses on nursing administration or nursing management for those who are majoring in these fields. It could also serve as a supplemental reference in nurse practitioner programs as well as in courses identified as structures and services in nursing or health care delivery systems. It might be appropriate in graduate nursing programs where the major is nursing administration and supervision but the theoretical material is presented by a graduate school of business. In these cases, a nursing orientation is often reinforced through a practicum-discussion led by a nurse, and this text might be useful for the discussion.

Furthermore, this text might be suitable as a basic or supplemental reference for allied health professionals who are majoring in the delivery or administration of health care services. It could also be used by those who design continuing education courses or inservice programs to help graduate nurses become more effective managers.

At whatever level the text is used, the nurse-learner must have already mastered the basic skills of nursing. Therefore, the text would be appropriate for an upper level baccalaureate course, an inservice course for graduate nurses moving toward leadership positions, or a graduate nursing course at the master's level.

ACKNOWLEDGMENTS

We wish to thank our students who stimulated our interest in the need for this book; also, Shirley Smoyak, Suzanne Hawes, and Sally Barhydt who encouraged its development; Marianne Peters whose clerical assistance made it possible; and our families—Bill and John, Deirdre, and Maura who shared our involvement and gave us time to accomplish our work.

Carolyn Chambers Clark
Carole A. Shea

Part One

Management: Theory and Process

This section presents basic system concepts and management processes that can be applied in a variety of health care systems. Systems theory provides a dynamic view of the organizational environment of health care. Management is the linking process that allows nurses to deliver quality care in organizational settings by interfacing with subsystems of the organization.

Chapter 1 identifies the conceptual framework for the chapters that follow. Management is examined from a systems viewpoint. System is defined and examples related to nursing and health care delivery are given. Management is defined and ways in which the manager links together subsystems are presented. Finally, a rationale for studying management from a systems stance is presented.

Chapter 2 discusses the following aspects of the organizational environment: traditional and system approaches to organizations, formal and informal structures of the organization, the advantages and disadvantages of centralized and decentralized authority, the difference between staff and line positions, guidelines for analyzing the quality of the organizational climate, types of leadership styles and examples of when each might be appropriate, and the hospital as an organization.

Chapter 3 defines the planning process; discusses how to choose objectives; suggests what nurse-managers might consider when planning or examining a budget; suggests ways to use time and plan staffing; explores guidelines for decision making, problem solving, and information-exchange interviews; and identifies task and maintenance behaviors that can permit managers to exert leadership.

Chapter 4 examines some of the quantitative tools used in decision-making and suggests ways in which the nurse-manager could work with an operations researcher to quantify the decision-making process. Some of the tools that could be of value to nurse-managers in this area include probability theory, sampling theory, linear programming, queuing theory, inventory theory, computer use, hospital models, simulation, network scheduling, and participative forecasting.

Chapter 5 examines the evaluation process from a home health agency perspective. Evaluation is defined and the appropriate objectives are examined. An example of this process in one community agency is presented. Utilization review and staff performance appraisal are also discussed.

Chapter 1

Management from a Systems Viewpoint

Carolyn Chambers Clark and Carole A. Shea

OBJECTIVES

After studying this chapter, the learner will:

- Define system
- Define management
- Define health care system
- Tell why nurses study systems and management

DEFINITION OF A SYSTEM

A system is an organized whole that is composed of interactive subsystems. Wholeness means that a system does not behave as a composite of its parts, but as a coherent, inseparable entity. In this respect, the whole is more than the sum of its parts. Each part or subsystem can effect change in all other parts and in the total system (Watzlawick 1967, p. 123). Also, a change can be initiated from outside that system (the external environment). For example, illness in a family member affects the entire family system by changing roles and functions related to activities of daily life. Likewise, an economic recession can influence family system functioning. Almost any change or innovation has ramifications for other parts of an open system (Miller 1965, p. 200).

Subsystems are separated from one another and from the larger system by boundaries. A closed system has rigid boundaries that permit minimal, if any, exchange with the external environment. Closed systems are nonhuman, mechanistic entities. Examples of closed systems in the health care field are problem-oriented records, wheelchairs, and unit dose medications. An open system has flexible boundaries that allow a dynamic interchange with the external environment or suprasystem. Open systems are biological and social and are in a continual state of change. Examples of open systems are living cells, nurse-doctor relationships, and health care planning committees.

The open or closed state of a system is dependent to some degree on the frame of reference used. It is possible to think of open properties in closed systems and closed properties in open systems. Medications may react chemically to the air or to other substances, record systems can be changed by human interaction and vice versa, and nurse-doctor communication in one hospital may be relatively free and open while in another setting may be formal and indirect. Openness or closedness of a boundary is controlled from both sides "as in the case of a door between adjoining hotel rooms that can be locked or unlocked on either side" (Hearn 1976, p. 29). A condition of complete openness or closedness is only possible when there is agreement about the definition of the boundary. Conflict is the result of openness on one side of a social system and closedness on the other (Hearn 1976, p. 29).

Interface is the point of contact of one system with another (Kast and Rosenzweig, 1974, p. 114). A hospital system has interfaces with many other systems: consumers; other health care agencies; local, state, and federal governmental agencies; drug and equipment companies; schools of nursing and medicine; and employment agencies or prospective employees. There are transfers of energy, people, money, information, and materials at various interfaces. In the case of an increase in the staff/client ratio due to such events as the opening of a new hospital unit or a large industrial accident, personnel can be employed from outside the system or deployed within the system to reestablish equilibrium. Thus, money and people are transferred at the interface between prospective employees and a health care system or within a health care system.

These transfers allow for dynamic equilibrium and adaptation to the external environment through the continuous exchange of energy, material, and information. Equilibrium is a dynamic state in which energies are used to repair and maintain the system as well as to change the structure of the system. Massive environmental changes may produce a crisis in which the person, group, or organization is unable to adapt. Dynamic equilibrium or steady state is then disrupted. This could occur if funds are inadequate to hire necessary personnel or if absenteeism prohibits effective triage. Systems cannot remain in disequilibrium indefinitely. The steady state is regained by reorganization of the structure and processes of its subsystems to the previous level or to a higher level of functioning.

Feedback is a concept that relates to changes within a system. In feedback, "part of the system's output is reintroduced into the system as information about the output" (Barry 1972, p. 184). When feedback is appropriate, the system's stability and adaptation are more likely to be assured. In this way, steady state is maintained by a circular, dynamic, and continuous process. Positive feedback leads to change and adaptation; negative feedback maintains steady state and enables the system to have stable relationships (Watzlawick 1967, p. 30).

The input of a social system (or organization) includes energy, people, money, materials, and information. In one form, information is a signal to the system about how it is functioning. The system can accept or reject this signal. Open systems are more receptive to new information, whereas closed systems are more likely to reject the signal. Throughput, the activity of an organization or system, includes such behaviors as client care, teaching, research, and maintenance of the system. The output of a system consists of services, products, and rewards to the people or subsystems of the organization. A system, then, can be conceptualized in terms of input⟶throughput⟶output, with a circular, feedback loop.

All systems have a hierarchy of components (Bertalanffy 1952). Biologically, cells are organized into tissues, tissues are organized into organs, and so on. Socially, people are organized into groups, groups are organized into departments, and so on. With increasing complexity, order is needed to coordinate activities or processes. For this purpose, subsystems are clustered or combined in a hierarchical structure. They are arranged in levels that bring together the parts of the whole along some dimension such as authority, educational preparation, influence, experience, or the goals and needs of the organization. A hierarchical structure has the shape of a pyramid. A hospital organization has an administrator at the top, a few managers or supervisors at the middle level, and many health care providers and consumers at the bottom.

In a systems frame of reference, there is no direct cause-and-effect relationship. Final states can be reached from different starting points along various pathways. This property of systems is called equifinality. Smoyak gives an example of this property in her description of employee turnover in nursing. She lists the following conditions that may lead to the final state of leaving: pregnancy, husband's transfer, family pressure, entering school, and dissatisfaction with nursing (Smoyak 1976, p. 221).

DEFINITION OF MANAGEMENT

Systems theory concepts provide the foundation for developing a view of management that considers the interaction between people and the organization in the context of the larger society. Management is the process of linking together individuals or work groups around specific problems or issues of the work environment (Bennis 1966). The management process uses both interpersonal and technical skills to achieve organizational objectives by utilizing human and material resources and technology (Longest 1976, p. 38). According to the systems approach, the management process has inputs of people, money, equipment, materials, and energy that are transformed to meet the organizational objectives (outputs) such as products or services rendered. Management is the essential activity to maintain a functioning organization (Stevens 1976, p. 44).

Management and administration are two terms that are often used interchangeably. The difference between management and administration has to do with the scope of executive functions, not the nature of the functions; administration has a broader scope or greater number of functions (Stevens 1976, p. 37). Administration is more comprehensive and includes such executive activities as setting goals and formulating policy, as well as managing personnel and materials. Thus, a director of nursing is an administrator who sets goals, formulates policy, and manages the nurses who provide care, or, in some institutions, participates in these decision-making processes with other departmental administrators on behalf of the nursing department. Nursing supervisors, head nurses, and even staff nurses participate in the management process according to their position in the organizational hierarchy.

This linking process of management has five important functions: planning, organizing, directing, controlling, and coordinating human and physical resources. The planning function includes deciding what to do in advance and how to do it. Short-, medium-, and long-term objectives, methods, and procedures are chosen, based on organizational constraints. Planning can be done on many levels in the system. Nursing care plans, team assignments, vacation schedules, department budgets, and institutional certificates-of-need exemplify five different levels of planning. Planning is continuous and the most important management function because it overlaps with all other functions (Longest 1976, p. 42).

The organizing function implies the integration of people and their activities as a cohesive unit that is focused on the goals of the organization. This entails a cooperative effort by a team of coworkers. It is important to understand interpersonal relationships, as well as how to decrease conflict and anticipate problems. For example, the professional nurse organizes the care of a client according to the assessed needs of that client and the proficiency of the available nursing staff.

Once the preparatory functions of planning and organizing have been effected, the manager concentrates on the directing function—communicating to the workers what work must be done. The most important aspect of directing is the initiation of action—putting the plan into operation according to the way the work has been organized. Directing includes the following activities: order-giving, supervising, leading, motivating, and communicating (Longest, 1976, p. 45). Communication, verbal and/or nonverbal, can include verbal change-of-shift reports, written assignment sheets, doctors' orders, informal commands, and policy directives from the administration. In exercising the directing function, the manager has the complex task of meshing the personal objectives of individuals and groups of individuals with the organization's objectives.

Coordination links together the various participants and channels their activities toward the achievement of mutual organizational goals. This process requires the simultaneous interaction among different departments and a high degree of labor specialization. Coordination is synchronization to produce a minimum of conflict and a maximum of collaboration among organization members. When coordination fails or is inadequate, conflict results. Some conflict may be healthy as a stimulus for change. However, the manager attempts to contain and resolve conflict by means of the coordinating function, using the mechanisms of the organization's hierarchy, the administrative system, and certain voluntary activities of the members. A collaborative effort that uses teams, task forces, committees, and persons designated as coordinators can accomplish something that is far greater than the sum of its individual parts.

In all organizations the control function is essential. Directly linked to the planning function, control is the regulation of activities in an organization so that what is planned is actually accomplished. This means the measurement and corrective action of persons and things to ensure that objectives and goals are reached according to plan. Control techniques include three steps: establishing standards, measuring performance and comparing the actual results with the standards, and correcting deviations from the standards (Longest, 1976, p. 49). In the delivery of health care, control of the quality of care at the lowest cost is of high priority. Examples of the controlling process include nursing audit, peer review, and development of outcome criteria.

Taken together, the five management functions form a managerial subsystem in the larger organization system. An effective manager must be able to perform all these functions. "The managerial subsystem spans the entire organization by relating the organization to its environment, setting goals, developing comprehensive, strategic, and operational plans, designing the structure, and establishing control processes" (Kast and Rosenzweig 1974, p. 113). Thus, the manager performs these functions simultaneously in an integrative relation to the other subsystems of the organization (Figure 1-1).

DEFINITION OF A HEALTH CARE SYSTEM

Defining "health care system" is difficult because health itself has not been quantified. DeGreene (1976, p. 293) insists that there may be no system at all, but merely bits and pieces of care. Arriving at a definition is further complicated by the inability of those involved to agree on the goals of a health care system and to make quantitative definitions.

One way to define health care system is to list and describe the levels or subsystems of client services within the organization or suprasystem. Six subsystems have been singled out for discussion. The one that is the weakest link in the health care system is preventive care (*Trends affecting the U.S. health care system* 1976, p. 263); this includes both education and prevention. Provider groups are school health education programs, well-baby clinics, family planning clinics, poison information and control centers, the American Health Foundation, and various governmental programs such as the National Center for Disease Control.

Another subsystem is primary care, which includes early detection and routine care. Provider groups are hospital outpatient departments, school and college health units, industrial health units, and community health centers. Preventive and primary care may be integrated through neighborhood health centers, migrant health centers, and office-based doctor practices.

A third subsystem is secondary or acute care, which includes critical care and emergency treatment. Provider groups are hospital emergency services, ambulatory services for clients where hospital equipment is used, and inpatient services in medical and surgical hospitals.

Tertiary care or special care is another subsystem of health care; this means highly technical services for clients in a large geographic area. Provider groups include specialty hospitals and general hospitals with highly specialized facilities. Teaching hospitals act as integrators for these two subsystems.

Another subsystem, restorative care, includes immediate follow-up care, rehabilitation, and home care. Provider groups are homes for unwed mothers; halfway houses for psychiatric clients; home health agencies;

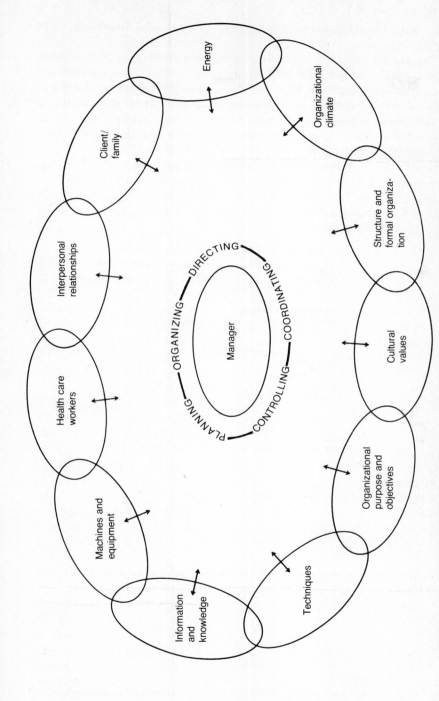

Figure 1-1 The manager links together subsystems of the organization.

9

and progressive care, extended care, rehabilitation, and home care units in hospitals.

The last subsystem is continuing care. Long-term care, chronic care, and personal care are provided in personal care homes, domicilary homes, inpatient health facilities for the mentally retarded or disturbed, and geriatric care centers. Examples of integration between restorative care and continuing care include nursing homes; health facilities for those with alcohol and drug abuse problems; and health facilities for the deaf, blind, and physically handicapped (*Trends* 1976, p. 262).

Health care systems are sociotechnical and social systems. They are just one unit in a suprasystem that includes education, welfare, economy, insurance, migration, urban affairs, environment, transportation, and scientific and technological advances. Each part of the suprasystem interfaces with the health care system (Figure 1-2).

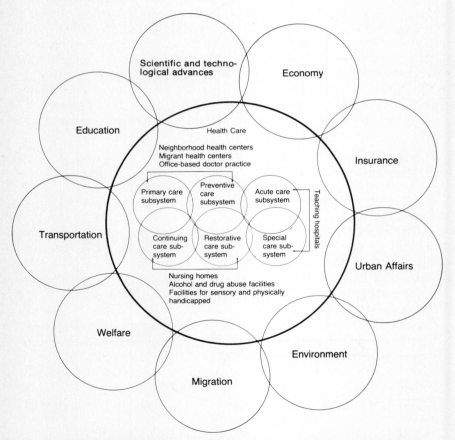

Figure 1-2   The health care system interfaces with other systems of the suprasystem.

The health care system in this country is vast and diffuse. At times, hospitals and professional health-givers try to discourage coordination of system elements. Traditionally, coordination of patient care has been based largely on fragmented physician referral systems (*Trends* 1976, p. 286). Thus, there have been omissions and duplications of effort. Furthermore, consumers are confused about how and where to enter the health care system. Health Maintenance Organizations (HMOs) and other interinstitutional referrals are beginning to make inroads into the inefficient and often discriminatory doctor referral system (*Trends* 1976, p. 287).

The health care system gives top priority to acute care and low priority to preventive and continuing care. Competition for clients occurs among doctors, and consumers have little voice in determining the kind of hospital care they receive (*Trends* 1976, p. 261).

Leininger (1973, pp. 171–173) has proposed an ''open client-centered health care system model'' as an alternative to the present arrangement. Her system includes more community-based health assessment. The consumer group would define wellness, and each client would choose the professional with whom to work. There would be major emphasis on health maintenance through prevention and restoration. Nurses (and other professional workers) would be prepared to function in either the wellness or illness subsystems. Leininger's model emphasizes distributed authority and control and individual responsibility. Since Leininger's model is simply a proposed system, nurses need to become familiar with what exists at present.

REASONS WHY NURSES STUDY SYSTEMS AND MANAGEMENT

King (1976, pp. 51–53) points out that a systems approach is needed in nursing because of the great complexity of nursing situations. According to her, nursing tasks may change over time, but the nursing decision-making function will remain. Systems theory offers a way to organize and study elements that interact with one another and that are related. King believes that nurses need to consider three interacting systems: the personal or individual system (intrapersonal); the group (interpersonal); and the society or social system, such as the hospital or the community.

Howland (1976, p. 121) takes a larger systems view. He states that the problems of managing health systems can no longer be solved by looking only at subsystems such as the nurse-client interaction. From his view, the total system and the components or subsystems in interaction must be studied.

Hearn (1976, pp. 61–68) describes systems interventions by social workers that can be useful to nurses, too. The potential for client dependency can be decreased by redistributing the energy of the helper-helpee relationship. For example, the nurse can enable the client to help others by teaching them, assisting them, participating in self-help groups, and so on. This intervention lessens the possibility of a never ending dependency of the client on the helper. The nurse can provide boundary maintenance by helping to delineate boundaries, regulating inputs, and varying the openness and closedness of the boundaries as necessary. Within the nurse-client subsystem, the use of counseling skills and physical exercise techniques can help clients define their intrapersonal and interpersonal boundaries. When the client is threatened, the boundaries need to be clearly defined by the nurse. The nurse can help the client to define boundaries clearly by means of summary statements, verbal directives, anxiety-reducing measures, and provision of basic needs. The nurse regulates the system inputs and outputs by providing appropriate feedback, performing treatments, and increasing or decreasing sensory stimulation. Systems can be encouraged to define their boundaries by regulating the degree of openness and closedness; the nurse can help to regulate openness and closedness of sensory and intellectual-emotional boundaries by assisting clients in testing reality and solving problems. The nurse can also help the client by using system concepts to provide the resources of people, materials, and ideas.

In order to make informed decisions, the nurse decision-maker needs to be able to assess the consequences for any alteration in the system. Sills (1976, p. 177) gives the example of a pharmacy department (subsystem) that develops a new method for drug administration and how this will affect the interface with the subsystem of nursing.

Rosen (1976, pp. 73–79) focuses on the administrative subsystem whose goal is control. The administrator coordinates subsystems to attain organizational goals. Control is initiated via the traditional power bases of reward and punishment, and is augmented by the power of expertise or by receiving power from other people. Systems concepts can help the nurse to identify interacting subsystems of power and control (such as the medical staff and the hospital administrator) as well as interacting contradictory role expectations of the nurse, doctor, administrator, and consumer. Systems concepts, then, can help the nurse organize highly complex data, make appropriate decisions, and intervene at the subsystem or system level. Interfaces between systems are also available for nursing intervention after considering all aspects of the system.

The management of health care delivery systems is of major concern to health care providers and consumers alike. Longest (1976, p. 1) describes a paradox created by health care today; despite the dramatic increase in medical knowledge, technology, and clinical proficiency, there is a growing dissatisfaction among client-provider subsystems with health care delivery. Professional health care providers have to pay attention to the management of delivery systems because there is pressure from various social groups for more and better services at lower costs. Traditionally, health professionals have not been educated and trained in management concepts, although they frequently occupy management positions. This is particularly true of nurses who have always managed care, as well as other nurses and personnel (as nurses or supervisors) without the benefit of formal education in management. Today, health professionals have to learn how to practice professionally in an organizational context that requires the use of management skills because most health care is delivered in complex organizational settings or interfaces with such organizations (Longest 1976, p. 3). These organizations include hospitals, clinics, community health agencies, nursing homes, HMOs, and group practices that provide professionals with supportive skills, technology, information, and physical resources. In an effort to provide quality care, professionals must learn to work effectively within the organization system and realistically consider economic and environmental constraints.

SUMMARY

A system is an organized whole composed of interactive subsystems. Systems theory concepts include wholeness, boundaries, openness and closedness, interface, dynamic equilibrium, feedback loop, hierarchy, and equifinality. Examples are drawn from the health care system to describe systems concepts as they pertain to organization and management.

Management is the process of linking together individuals or work groups around specific problems or issues of the work environment. This linking process has five major functions that the manager performs: planning, organizing, directing, coordinating, and controlling. Health professionals have to use management skills in order to deliver quality care in organizational settings.

Health care systems are difficult to define because health itself has not been quantified. However, one way to define a health care system is according to levels or subsystems of client services within the organization or suprasystem. The six levels of the health care system are: (1) preventive care, (2) primary care, (3) secondary or acute care, (4) tertiary or special care, (5) restorative care, and (6) continuing care. Health care systems as sociotechnical and social systems are part of the suprasystem. Problems at entering the system, coordination of care, and priorities for care are discussed. Leininger's "open client-centered health care system model" is presented as an alternative to the diffuse health care system in existence today. Finally, the rationale for studying systems and management concepts is presented—to assist the nurse in providing quality care in an organizational context and its interfaces.

REFERENCES

Barry, M. Patricia. 1972. Feedback concepts in family therapy. *Perspectives in Psychiatric Care* 10,4:183–189.

Bennis, Warren. 1966. *Beyond bureaucracy: essays on the development and evolution of human organizations.* New York: McGraw-Hill.

Bertalanffy, Ludwig von. 1952. *Problems of life: an evaluation of modern biological thought.* New York: Wiley.

———. 1966. General systems theory and psychiatry. *American handbook of psychiatry.* Vol. 3. New York: Basic Books.

———. 1976. Introduction. In *Health research: the systems approach,* ed. Harriet H. Werley, Ann Zuzich, Myron Zajkowski, and A. Dawn Zagornik. New York: Springer, pp. 5–14.

Clements, Imelda W.; and Buchanan, Dianne. 1976. The use of analogies in introducing the systems concepts to families in therapy. In *The psychiatric nurse as a family therapist,* ed. Shirley Smoyak. New York: Wiley, pp. 24–29.

DeGreene, Kenyon B. 1976. Concepts and problems in the test and evaluation of health systems. In *Health research: the systems approach,* ed. Harriet H. Werley, Ann Zuzich, Myron Zajkowski, and A. Dawn Zagornik. New York: Springer, pp. 293–313.

Leininger, Madeleine. 1973. Open client-centered health care system model. *Nursing Outlook* 73,3:171–173.

Longest, Beaufort. 1976. *Management practices for the health professional.* Reston, Va.: Reston Publishing.

Miller, J. G. 1965. Living systems: basic concepts. *Behavioral Science* 10:200.

Rizzo, Nicholas D. 1976. General system theory: its impact in the health fields. In *Health research: the systems approach,* ed. Harriet Werley, Ann Zuzich, Myron Zajkowski, and A. Dawn Zagornik. New York: Springer, pp. 12–24.

Smoyak, Shirley. 1976. Theories "produce" findings: studying effects of innovation in hospital nursing units. In *Health research: the systems approach,* ed. Harriet H. Werley, Ann Zuzich, Myron Zajkowski, and A. Dawn Zagornik. New York: Springer, pp. 215–224.

Stevens, Barbara J. 1975. *The nurse as executive.* Wakefield, Mass.: Contemporary Publishing.

———. 1976. *First line patient care management.* Wakefield, Mass.: Contemporary Publishing.

Trends affecting the U.S. health care system. 1976. Department of Health, Education and Welfare Publication No. HRA 76-14503. Washington, D.C.: U.S. Govt. Printing Office.

Watzlawick, P.; Beavin; J. H.; and Jackson, D. D. 1967. *Pragmatics of human communication.* New York: Norton.

Chapter 2

The Organizational Environment and Its Constraints

Carole A. Shea

OBJECTIVES

After studying this chapter, the learner will:

- Define organization using a systems framework
- Identify five components of the organizational environment
- Compare and contrast three organizational approaches to management
- Discuss a health agency's formal structure using an organizational chart
- List four advantages and four disadvantages of the informal structure
- Describe the effects of environmental constraints in terms of the health worker, the health agency, and the community

ORGANIZATIONAL ENVIRONMENT

Organizations are a way of life—inevitable and necessary for survival in a complex modern society. The delivery of most health care takes place in organizations that range in size from a large comprehensive medical center to a neighborhood drop-in clinic to a small group practice of independent practitioners. In order to influence health care delivery, nurses must understand how the organizational environment in which they work affects their nursing practice.

An organization is an open social system in which groups of people combine knowledge, techniques, skills, and resources to accomplish a goal-oriented task by integrating their structured activities. Organizations are people—people working in groups and using their knowledge and skills toward a goal (Kast and Rosenzweig 1974, p. 6). Examples of health care organizations include the World Health Organization, Planned Parenthood, HMOs, American Nurses Association, Medicare, Visiting Nurses Association, as well as certain universities and schools, hospitals, clinics, units in the military service, some religious orders, and special departments in the federal government.

Organizations do not exist in a vacuum; they encompass and are embedded in their environment. According to the systems view, the organization is an interdependent series of parts that include the physical plant, the individual workers, the formal structure, the informal work groups, the task, the management process, the organizational climate, styles of leadership, and other subsystems in the environment that directly and indirectly affect the organization (see Figure 1-1, p. 8). In addition to the internal subsystems of the organization, aspects of the operating process itself, such as communication, decision-making, and controlling mechanisms must be considered as they affect the organization and its environment. Lastly, the organization is influenced by the environment of the suprasystem that surrounds it, that is, persons, groups, other organizations, and forces beyond the boundary of the organization system itself that require a response from the organization (Schaefer 1975, p. 15). The suprasystem might be the local community, the regional HSA, an international business conglomerate, or the Department of Health, Education and Welfare.

The relationship between an organization and its environment is characterized by organizational behavior that is *responsive* or *effective* to its environment (Metcalfe 1976, p. 328). Environmental responsiveness means that an organization changes its policies and procedures in order to accommodate itself to external conditions. Environmental effectiveness means that an organization attempts to modify the environment in order to obtain inputs of resources and people that are more congruent with its objectives. Most organizations use the responsiveness mode in relating to their environment. For example, a hospital may respond to a cutback in its share of federal monies by decreasing the number of professional nurses on its staff, thereby vitiating its objective to provide high quality nursing care for its clients. Internal standards are compromised in response to external pressures. Responsiveness causes a problem when organizational objectives must continually be reconciled with external expectations (Metcalfe 1976, p. 329). Because environmental factors are rapidly changing, and less attention has been directed toward modifying external demands, health organizations often have difficulty maintaining a continuity of policy and goals. For instance, some health agencies operate according to management by crisis rather than according to management by objectives. This is more likely to be the case in such organizations as a large city hospital. There, the work of the system cannot be mechanized, standardized, or preplanned, since one has little control over the volume or makeup of the workload at any given time (Georgopoulos 1976, p. 18). As a result, the hospital organization tries to stabilize its equilibrium by organizing its internal environment along rigid hierarchical lines with greater administrative controls (Smith 1972, p. 23). However, this rigidity further diminishes the possibility of developing new responsive and effective behaviors. Instead, the organization allows the requirements of the hierarchical structure to dictate ready-made slots into which people and resources must fit. When this situation exists, the organization cannot hire a clinical nurse specialist because there is no such designated position on the organizational chart. Such organizational behavior demonstrates a lack of positive environmental responsiveness in its inability to use creatively this new resource.

The organizational environment includes the organization entity with its subsystems and the operating process, as well as the suprasystem in which it exists. In order to analyze certain components of these systems, the nurse-manager needs to understand how people work and how the organization operates. There is no universally accepted organization theory that explains the behavior of people in their world of work. However, since the 1900s, several approaches to organization and management have been developed that have influenced the leaders and managers in today's organizations. Of these, the traditional, the human relations, and the systems approaches will be discussed.

ORGANIZATIONAL APPROACHES

Traditional

The traditional approach to organizational management, called scientific management, was developed by Frederick Taylor, an engineer who wanted to find the one best way to do a particular job. He gave primary emphasis to planning, standardizing, and improving human efforts at the operative level in order to maximize output with a minimum of input.

The planning of work was separated from the performance; executives at the top devised the work plan that workers carried out although they had no say in the plan, the method, or the working conditions. The manager's main task was to supervise and control subordinates in their specialized jobs. The workers were expected to be motivated by economic rewards to achieve higher productivity (Kast and Rosenzweig 1974, p. 55). In general, managers in companies using a scientific management approach tried to structure the organization, formalize relationships, and establish rules and procedures to maximize efficient productivity.

Another contributor to the traditional approach was Henri Fayol, who believed that management was a universal function that could be defined in terms of a management process. He said that every manager must plan, organize, command, coordinate, and control. Fayol's fourteen principles, such as division of work, scalar chain, and centralization were meant to be guidelines for managers to use in designing an organization's structure (Kast and Rosenzweig 1974, pp. 58–59). Although Fayol's work has been modified; it continues to influence modern organizations.

Max Weber, a German sociologist and contemporary of Taylor and Fayol, developed the bureaucratic model to represent an ideal organizational structure. Today, the term "bureaucracy" connotes red tape, inefficency, and frustrating officials. Originally the bureaucratic structure was intended as a rational regulation of power. Weber's bureaucracy is characterized by (Longest 1976, pp. 109–110):

1   A clear-cut division of labor with a high degree of specialization of functions.

2   Positions arranged in a hierarchy so that each lower office is under the supervision and control of a higher office.

3   A consistent system of abstract rules and regulations to ensure uniformity and coordination.

4   Impersonal relationships with workers to prevent unfair treatment or undue advantage.

5   Technical competence as the basis for selecting a person for a position or promotion.

Bureaucracies in the abstract are rational, efficient, stable, and durable. In practice, bureaucratic organizations are often rigid, inflexible, resistant to change, and dehumanizing. However, all complex organizations use some features of bureaucratic design to administer and manage policies, people, and products efficiently and productively.

Criticism of the traditional approach and the bureaucratic model focuses on the treatment of workers like cogs in a well-oiled machine, without regard for their individuality and complex motivation. Both the external environmental factors and the internal ones are discounted as if the organization were a closed system (Kast and Rosenzweig 1974, pp. 70–71). The more closely an organization adheres to this traditional approach, the more likely that people's work experience will be dehumanizing.

Human Relations

Traditional approaches emphasized the need for order, stability, and authority based on scientific principles without regard for the human element—the people in the organization. In response to criticisms of the traditional perspective, the human relations approach was developed. The Hawthorne studies of the 1930s demonstrated the importance of human resources and informal group relationships to the overall functioning of an organization. While accepting the structural aspects of traditional organization, reformers changed the thinking about the human element in organizations. They pointed to social and psychological factors as having a major impact on worker satisfaction and productivity. The manager tried to build morale by making each worker feel useful and a participant in management decision making; the workers were to have input in executive planning. It was assumed that individual goals and needs were more important than money in motivating people to work (Claus and Bailey 1977, p. 122). Douglas McGregor described people's motivation to work in terms of his theory X and theory Y. Theory X says that management consists of getting things done through other people (McGregor 1972, p. 118). This theory assumes that the average person dislikes work, lacks ambition, dislikes responsibility, wants to be led, is indifferent to the organization's needs, is resistant to change, is self-centered, and is gullible. Theory Y is the opposite of theory X. It says that the essential task of management is to arrange organizational conditions and methods of operation so that people can best achieve their own goals by directing their efforts toward organizational objectives (McGregor, p. 122). Theory Y assumes that people like to work, can direct and control their actions, will seek and enjoy responsibility, can achieve personal goals simultaneously with organizational goals, and will live up to the high expectations of others (Stevens 1975, p. 33). Theory Y is consistent with the human relations approach, while theory X typifies the underlying assumptions of the traditional approach.

While human values in organizations must be considered, critics of the human relations approach say that there is too much emphasis on the psychosocial aspects to the detriment of organizational efficiency and productivity. Human relations techniques, which imply participation and some measure of democracy, actually do nothing to change the basic power structure or to challenge the manager's right to control because the hierarchical structure is still there (Bucklow 1973, p. 462). Also, the human relations approach has tended to view the organization as a closed system without regard for environmental, economic, and political influences and constraints (Kast and Rosenzweig 1974, p. 82).

Systems

The traditional approach tried to separate activities into fragmented tasks and operational units. The human relations approach dealt with motivations and relationships. Neither approach gives sufficient emphasis to the integration and coordination of activities and interrelationships in a complex organizational system (Kast and Rosenzweig 1974, p. 109). Those who adopt a modern approach study organizations as systems of mutually dependent parts and variables; the organization is perceived as a social system within the suprasystem of society. Modern organization theory and general systems theory share many of the same concepts, and both view the organization as an integrated whole. Accordingly, the organization is seen as a dynamic system that is (1) divided into units that interact with one another and with the environment, (2) structured to maintain information flow and communication, (3) assured of growth and viability, and (4) required to have integrated and effective decision-making processes (Kast and Rosenzweig 1974, pp. 109–114). The organization is an open system that interacts continually with its environment. Attention is focused on the process of guiding the organizational output rather than on the rational structure or social process of the organization (Arnold 1968, pp. 10, 24). Management concepts have shifted from ideas about individual roles and positions to the dynamic interchange within a system and with its environment.

This systems approach poses a difficult and complex assignment for the nurse-manager who must attempt to understand the organization as a system, recognize the relationships between subsystems, and integrate the parts in working toward the organizational goal. Those within the organization are affected simultaneously by the constraints exacted by a rapidly changing environment and the internal forces—people, politics, and resources—of the organization. The worker in a modern organization should have a systems orientation, a mind that "integrates disparate facts into a creative whole . . . [and] asks questions in order to test a hypothetical model in his head rather than making a list to later analyze and make sense of" (Maccoby 1976, p. 81).

The systems approach to management is comprehensive and complex because problem solving is based on examining interacting variables rather than discrete, causal relationships. Knowledge from the physical, biological, and social sciences is integrated to provide a framework for understanding organizations within an increasingly unstable environment.

ORGANIZATIONAL STRUCTURE

Having some idea of what an organizational environment is, one needs to understand how an organization is structured. Structure is the means by which an organization attempts to achieve its purpose, philosophy, and objectives. Organizational structure refers to the grouping of positions and the establishment of patterns of relationships among the organization's parts (Kast and Rosenzweig 1974, p. 207). It specifies which persons in these positions are to perform which types of work, and it coordinates all activities of the organization (Price et al. 1974, p. 29). Davis says that structure focuses on the job and not the people who do it. This is significant because the structure partly determines the people's power and their perceptions of their roles (Davis 1972, pp. 197, 212). Organizational structure, or the pattern of behavior and relationships in organizations, is relatively stable and slow to change.

Formal Structure

Organizations have both a formal and an informal structure. The formal structure is a deliberate plan or blueprint that relates people and their tasks to the work environment in order to help the organization attain its objectives. It includes the pattern of formal relationships and duties designated in the organizational chart and the job descriptions, as well as the formal rules, policies, procedures, control mechanisms, and compensation arrangements of the organization (Kast and Rosenzweig 1974, p. 208). The informal structure is the network of social and personal relationships that arise spontaneously and inevitably as a result of people working together, without the sanction of formal authority. Formal structure emphasizes positions in terms of authority and function; informal structure emphasizes people and their relationships (Davis 1972, p. 252).

Formal structure as one component of the organization system should be varied to suit the purpose, the people, the task, and the work environment. No one design is best for all organizations. When the work is more routinized, such as in an automobile assembly plant, the structure may be a fixed, hierarchical model. However, work that is complex and varied, such as nursing care, requires a more open, flexible structure allowing for open communication and professional autonomy. The choice of a particular structure must be determined by the type of work, the building and location, financial resources, equipment and supplies, technology, and the availability and expertise of the people who must be organized to deliver effective, efficient, and economical goods and services (Beyers and Phillips 1971, p. 8). In the case of a hospital, the nature of the work—client care, teaching, research, and prevention—precludes the use of a single structure for all departments. For example, the x-ray department may be hierarchically structured, while the research laboratory may have a matrix organization.

Authority, Responsibility, Accountability

Authority is one of the major patterned relationships established according to the formal structure. Authority is the right to act or to command the action of others based on one's formal position in an organization and one's control of sanctions and rewards. Formal authority comes with the position and is not vested in the person. For example, Head Nurse Brown has legitimate authority over Staff Nurse Jones because he or she is in the Head Nurse position and not because of any personal influence. If Staff Nurse Jones is delegated the position of Acting Head Nurse in Mr. or Ms. Brown's absence, he or she would have the power and authority that goes with the position. However, the power to command is meaningless unless the subordinate accepts the obligations of the assignment, that is, acts with responsibility to complete the task assigned. By accepting the responsibility or not, the subordinate controls the response to authority (Davis 1972, p. 200). Delegation refers to the act of management of assigning tasks together with the authority necessary to accomplish the job. A superior can delegate authority but not responsibility, which requires the active acceptance by the subordinate. Linked with the delegation of authority and the assumption of responsibility is the concept of accountability for the overall process. Accountability means that the subordinate is both answerable and liable to the superior for the quality and quantity of the assigned task, and the superior is accountable for delegating the proper activity to the appropriate person and for his or her own acts (Price et al. 1974, p. 21). Accountability, like responsibility, cannot be delegated. Issues of authority, responsibility, and accountability are important to the nursing community. Nurses have traditionally assumed a lot of responsibility but have lacked the delegated authority to put "muscle" into their professional practice. Recent changes in authority patterns have called for increased accountability among nurses who are striving to utilize the increased authority with the responsibility to deliver professional nursing care.

Organization Chart

An organization chart diagrams the planned arrangement of people, indicates various positions and their relationships to one another, and specifies formal authority and communication networks (see Figure 2-1). This two-dimensional, abstract model of an organizational structure usually takes the form of a hierarchical pyramid. The hierarchy is based on the scalar principle in which there is a vertical division or scale of duties

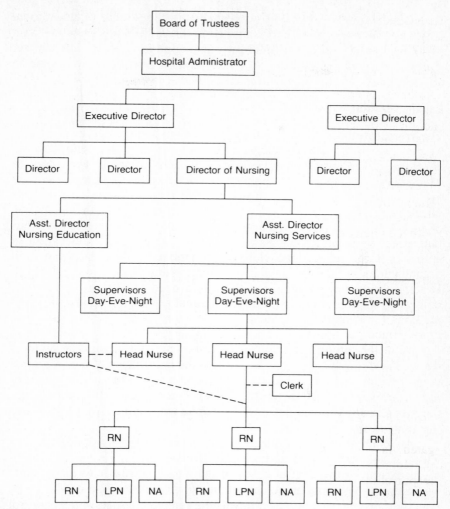

Figure 2-1 A traditional hospital organization chart.

into levels with functional units according to degrees of authority and responsibility (Davis 1972, p. 197). Traditionally decision making and direction are executed at the top. Authority, responsibility, knowledge, and energy flow down the scalar chain, while accountability for the work and the methods of work flow up. On the chart, the title of each position generally indicates the work performed. The distance of a position from the top of the chart shows the relative status of that position. The lines between positions specify the established pattern for formal interactions and channels of communication. With job descriptions to clarify the positions, an organization chart presents a reasonable outline of the organizational structure. However, the chart is limited in that it does not show informal relationships, the degree of authority of a superior over a subordinate, interactions between equals, or lateral relationships between people in different parts of the organization (Kast and Rosenzweig 1974, p. 211).

Decentralization

The organizational structure determines the amount and degree of authority that can be delegated. Delegation of authority is either centralized or decentralized. Centralization is a management principle according to which planning and decision-making are done by a few people at the highest level in the hierarchy. Directives are communicated to workers through the formal chain of command. Decentralization is the delegation of authority to workers at the operational level, who then make decisions that affect their work. Douglass and Bevis believe that "delegation of authority to the agency level closest to the job to be done leads to overall organizational effectiveness and decision-making" (1974, pp. 109–112). In large, complex organizations there is a need for decentralization of control so that delegated authority can equal assumed responsibility and methods for communication can become more direct. This results in a more democratic sharing (participative management), with a decrease in control at the top and an increase of communication across hierarchical levels. Decentralization tends to increase the importance of the individual worker who is encouraged to make independent decisions and solve problems creatively and competently. However, the organization must maintain some control so that decentralized units will continue to work toward the goals of the organization.

An example of decentralization is the organization of nursing services within a hospital to shift authority for decision making related to direct client care from the central office of the nursing director to the bedside where the professional nurse delivers nursing care (see Figure 2-2). To be effective, decentralization also means the removal of hierarchical control and the reassignment of nonnursing functions (Simms 1973, p. 277). In planning for decentralization, one needs to consider the following factors (Mahowald 1974, p. 41):

1 The number of work groups.
2 The strength of ongoing relationships.
3 The combination of necessary skills held in common.
4 The number of personnel needed for staffing.
5 The best use of personnel.
6 The financial resources.

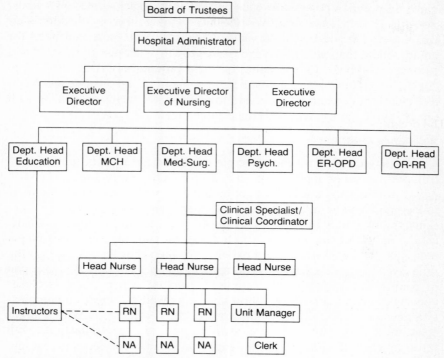

Figure 2-2   A decentralized nursing service.

The major clinical advantage of a decentralized system is that decision making is done by key nurse-managers who are proficient in their roles as clinical specialists or clinical coordinators (Stitely 1973, p. 250). Because of increased professional autonomy and personnel accountability, a two-way street is established so that nurses can communicate directly with and affect the decisions of the department head. Other advantages include increased job satisfaction among nurses; adaptability to rapid change; establishment of staff positions for nurses, such as inservice director and clinical coordinator; and a decrease in the operating budget because of the elimination of superfluous supervisors.

Decentralization can cause problems in an organization. Workers at the operational level may be incompetent or inadequately educated and trained to make good decisions. Good interpersonal relationships and complex communication skills may be in short supply. Departments may compete with one another and refuse to cooperate, thereby requiring more control and directives from top management. Overall objectives may be ignored or diverted as each unit attempts to achieve its own goals. Sometimes individual objectives actually sabotage the organization's effort to provide goods and services. Because of the increased need for coordination, there may be an excessive growth of service groups that add to the payroll but do not enhance efficient productivity (Davis 1972, pp. 222–223). An organization must be able to monitor the positive and negative effects of decentralization, and to develop the means for dealing with organizational stress and resistance to change.

Span of Control

Closely associated with the principle of decentralization is span of control, or the number of people one manager can effectively direct. The ratio of subordinates to superior cannot be fixed, but must reflect (1) the level in the organization (at a high level with many complex management functions, the ratio may be 5:1; at a low level where work is routinized, 15:1); (2) the nature of the work performed; (3) the capacity and skills of the manager; (4) the education and expertise of the subordinates; and (5) the time given to outside activities (Longest 1976, pp. 112–113). A small span of control indicates a tall hierarchical structure, where there is closer coordination and control of subordinates, as well as longer communication lines. The subordinate is likely to be "boss-oriented." With a larger span, there is a flatter structure (as in the case of decentralization), with fewer levels, diffusion of control, and many centers for decision making. There is less face-to-face contact between subordinates and their superior because there is more autonomy. Communication lines are shorter.

Organization size also affects the span of control. Larger companies generally prefer taller structures, and smaller companies, flatter structures. People have shown a preference for working in small organizations with flat structures. Studies have indicated that in large operating units there is less job satisfaction, more absenteeism, and a large turnover (Davis 1972, pp. 224–228). Nurses working in *small* hospital units might seem to be an exception to this generalization, since they demonstrate the same problems of job dissatisfaction, absenteeism, and turnover. One explanation for this is that quite often their immediate superior—the head nurse—lacks enough authority to make decisions for that unit, thus making that unit nonautonomous (Gaynor and Berry 1973, pp. 44–45). In effect, these staff nurses are not a small unit unto themselves but are really only a small part of the larger operating unit—the whole nursing department, which is ultimately under medical authority.

Line and Staff Positions

In complex organizations there is a need to integrate specialists and technological advances into the system. To facilitate this integration, the scalar principle of dividing duties into levels according to degrees of authority has been modified by the establishment of two types of organizational positions—line and staff. Line positions, connected by vertical lines on the organization chart, indicate lines of authority and accountability for those whose work pertains directly to achieving the organization's objectives. Staff positions are sometimes indicated by broken lines on the chart; there is no direct vertical connection between staff positions and line positions that are lower in the hierarchy. This indicates that people in staff positions have no formal authority over people in line positions. Instead, those in staff positions assist those in line positions, by lending expertise, helping in planning or research, or providing special services. Those in staff positions act in an advisory capacity but cannot command action from those in line positions. Staff positions in nursing are not the "staff nurses" who actually fill line positions. Inservice educators, nurse consultants, nurse coordinators, and some clinical specialists are in staff positions. However, without line authority, these advisory roles are often not as effective as they might be in instituting needed changes in traditional organizations (Price 1974, pp. 38–41).

Informal Structure

People often try to adjust the organizational structure to suit their personal as well as their work needs. In every organization, there is an informal structure that is not related to the formal structure. Relationships and interactions arise spontaneously that cut across the hierarchical levels and position lines. Because its emphasis is on people, not positions, the informal structure is not subject to control by the formal structure. Management must accept the fact that informal structure is inevitable, is composed of small groups whose members strongly influence one another, and has advantages as well as disadvantages (Longest 1976, p. 137).

The informal structure serves to perpetuate values, provide social satisfactions, disperse information, and exert control by influencing and regulating the behavior of the group members. Each of these purposes can be a potential area of difficulty for the organization's management (Davis 1972, pp. 254–257). The following instances exemplify common problems. Perpetuating values may mean a resistance to change. For example, the nurse who abides by the traditional role of "handmaiden to the doctor" will find it impossible to change his or her behavior in order to act as a professional colleague with the doctor. Seeking social satisfaction, the nurse may experience conflict about spending time talking with friends at work, rather than conversing with a sick client. Communication for the purpose of giving and getting information can degenerate into the passing on of unfounded rumors and gossip. Lastly, group pressures to control behavior may result in conformity or, in the case of the new graduate nurse, using unsafe techniques in order to avoid the derision and contempt for new ideas by older nurses who want to maintain the status quo.

The informal structure also has positive aspects. The informal structure is the "heart" of the organization, while the formal structure is the rational-legal "head." With only a formal structure, an organization's operation would be too inflexible and dogmatic to meet the needs of all the dynamic situations that arise daily. The informal structure permits and even encourages workers to "bend" the rules or make exceptions on certain occasions in order to expedite the organization's work objectives. Without the informal structure, an organization might seal its own doom because of its rigidity and strict adherence to the "letter of the law." For example, nurses often engage in activities that are not included in their job descriptions, such as client health teaching, family counseling, and community referrals. This extension of their roles allows needs to be met that might otherwise be ignored. To cite another instance, formal channels of communication may be circumvented in an emergency, such as when a staff nurse telephones a doctor at home in the middle of the night to report a sudden change in his or her client's medical condition, rather than spending time locating the night supervisor to report this information. Or, a young nurse may seek the advice of another nurse whose competence and knowledge he or she respects, rather than go to the designated team leader or supervisor whose manner may be less helpful or who may not be as approachable.

The informal structure also provides a sense of belonging and security to a small, cohesive group, and this tends to promote stability among the work force. This idea argues against the common practice of sending nurses to "float" on another ward that is short of nursing personnel. Such actions only contribute to the breakdown of cohesiveness and the lowering of morale.

A cooperative working group can make the manager's job easier because motivated workers who can be trusted require less supervision, and they may help to compensate for certain deficiencies in the manager's own skills. The head nurse of a primary nursing unit expects to do very little checking up to see that the client routines are carried out. Instead, his or her time can be much better spent in teaching new technology, conducting case study seminars, or instituting evaluation procedures such as a nursing audit. Often individual team members have expertise or a special facility for getting a job done quickly that the superior can rely upon.

Managers can also use the informal structure to determine their subordinates' feelings and attitudes by tuning into the grapevine (Longest 1976, pp. 142–143). This is a two-way communication in which the management can sound out the workers informally, and the workers can inform management of their problems and concerns without fear of reprisal. Rumors are the undesirable part of the grapevine; they are due to a combination of interest and ambiguity, and are usually incorrect. The best way to deal with harmful rumors is to seek out the cause of the rumor. Then, it is best for the manager to supply the facts in a face-to-face confrontation, followed by a confirmation in writing (Davis 1972, p. 269).

In essence, the informal structure makes the formal organization a workable venture, provided that management recognizes the existence and value of their interrelationships and tries to minimize any formal activities that unnecessarily threaten the informal groups.

Organizational Climate

Organizational climate refers to the "prevailing emotional state shared by members in the system; this may be formal, relaxed, defensive, cautious, accepting, trusting" (Dyer 1972, p. 176). The climate is created by managers and informal leaders who reflect their values regarding security, equity, respect for individual differences, and the development of potential skills and capabilities—a process of "humanizing work" (Maccoby 1976, p. 243). Ideally, the organizational climate should allow people to achieve maturity and dignity at their place of work. Four basic measures of perceived climate have been identified (Levenstein 1976, p. 53):

1 Individual autonomy—the degree to which the climate allows people to exercise freedom of action.

2 Structure—especially the organizational relationships through which leadership operates.

3 Rewards—both economic and psychological compensations geared to performance.

4 Consideration—the extent to which employees are treated as individuals.

In the past, health organizations have not provided a healthy climate for nurses: autonomy was denied; effective leadership was lacking; rewards were few; and the organization's needs were allowed to supersede those of the individual nurse, who was expected to be devoted to serving the needs of others (Brief 1976, p. 57).

Today, the climate is changing as nurses learn to assert their own rights and make more explicit both the role and the needs of the working nurse (Claus and Bailey 1976, pp. 38–39; Dyer 1972, p. 189). Walton's guidelines for analyzing the quality of the organizational climate in a nursing organization include (Claus and Bailey 1976, p. 38):

1 Compensation that is commensurate with the nurse's educational preparation, level of expertise, and fair market value.

2 Working conditions that provide for safe nursing practice and health maintenance of nurse and client.

3 Assignments that are challenging and make full use of the nurse's capabilities and talents.

4 Opportunities for continued professional and personal growth, and the assurance of security in the future.

5 Accordance of importance to individuals as part of the formal organization and valuing them as social members of the informal structure.

6 The guarantee and exercise of the nurse's constitutional rights and privileges in the organization.

7 The allowance of time for individual, family, and community activities.

8 Work that is scientifically significant, socially meaningful, and personally fulfilling.

Leadership

A crucial factor in the organizational climate is the leadership of managers who determine what the work atmosphere will be. Managers, by virtue of their formal position, can command people to take action. However, the most effective manager is the one who leads in such a way that subordinates want to cooperate in achieving the organization's objectives. O'Donovan defines leadership style as the way in which a manager "undertakes the processes of representation, interaction, standard setting, goal emphasis, participation, direction, rule enforcement, and motivation" (1975, p. 32). Leadership style is important because it affects the workers' morale and their productivity.

There are several different leadership styles; the most common ones described in the literature are autocratic (task-oriented) and democratic (relationship/people-oriented) (Heimann 1976, pp. 19–20). In positive terms, the autocrat is a highly competent person who makes good decisions. He or she works through and with people, controls individually, and uses personal influence. The autocrat first decides what needs to be done and then works hard to convince others to reach the same decision. To be effective, the autocrat must be sincere with the work group and willing to abide by the decisions of the group occasionally when the workers cannot be persuaded otherwise (O'Donovan 1975, p. 34). An ineffective autocrat is caricatured as a power-hungry, insensitive, dominating, and fear-inducing authoritarian. Mature, autocratic leadership is needed in nursing to provide direction and motivate nurses who are not used to participating in management functions and decision making.

A democratic leadership style is exemplified by the leader who looks to the group for direction, promotes cohesive group functioning, and trains others to assume leadership. The group is valued above the individual or the organization. Extremes of this approach may be harmful to the organization's efficiency because of the time-consuming nature of group decision making. Also, the personal interests of the group may interfere with or countermand the organization's goals. Subordinates may take unfair advantage of this type of leadership. However, if there are no abuses, nurses can benefit from this style of leadership. Nurses are often organized into teams where the leadership role is rotated or shared on a daily or weekly basis. The democratic style can develop leadership potential, collaborative skills, and collegial power.

Another style—known as laissez-faire—is really a lack of leadership. The laissez-faire leader gives information and materials to the work group, but does not give direction, exert control, or evaluate results. This tends to promote frustration, confusion, and dissatisfaction among the workers (Heimann 1976, pp. 20–21). There is no place in nursing for this no-leadership style. Even nurses who are practicing with professional autonomy need the direction, coordination, and motivation of good leadership.

Nurses need to adapt their leadership behavior to the work environment. In this sense, leadership is situation-specific. Effective leadership depends upon the appropriateness of the behavior in the work situation. According to Hersey, Blanchard, and LaMonica's life cycle theory of leadership, *how* leadership depends upon the situation, and *what* style is effective depends upon the relationship among three variables (Hersey, Blanchard, and La Monica 1976, p. 19):

1 The amount of direction (task behavior).
2 The amount of support (relationship behavior).
3 The maturity of the group (capacity to set high but attainable goals, willingness and ability to take responsibility, and the education and experience of the individual or group).

For example, a head nurse might use task behaviors in an autocratic style with a newly hired baccalaureate graduate. He or she might explain how, when, where, and what tasks must be done; define the goals of the organization; establish patterns for formal communication; and attempt to influence the nurse's perception of his or her role in the organization. With an older, more experienced staff nurse, the head nurse might focus on the relationship, giving emotional and psychological support, and facilitating professional behavior and personal growth. In providing leadership for a nursing aide, the head nurse might adopt behaviors that are both task-oriented and relationship-oriented. As the staff members become more skilled and proficient at their tasks, and as the social relationships promote cohesive group functioning, the work itself will require less task- and relationship-oriented behaviors and more facilitative and coordinative behaviors from the head nurse.

THE HOSPITAL ORGANIZATION

A hospital organization is more than a building, a place to work, a uniform, a community resource, or an educational institution. Georgopoulos has called the general hospital "a highly specialized and internally differentiated system which is intended to do certain work in order to solve particular human problems" (1972, p. 9). Well-managed hospitals are adaptive, sociotechnical systems composed of people who act, interact, communicate, think, feel, and make decisions in a purposeful way based on professional standards and the reflected needs of the community and its environment. With professional leadership, priorities and a healthy working order are established within the hospital. In turn, the organization can enhance the delivery of quality health care when its environment promotes autonomy and adherence to standards of professional behavior (Beyers and Phillips 1971, pp. 4–5). Hospitals are often prevented from reaching their full potential as professional, problem-solving systems by their organizational structure. The traditional hospital is a multilevel hierarchy with bureaucratic-like arrangements of positions and work assignments where authority resides at the top. Communication filters down rapidly from the top but is slow to rise up from the bottom. Decision-making is dominated by the power élites—the physicians, administrators, and trustees—who govern the organization and define the action framework for other health care workers and consumers (Georgopoulos 1972, p. 4). Nurses and clients, the largest of these groups, have little influence on decision making when the hospital is administered according to bureaucratic theory, which gives the least say to those at the bottom of the hierarchy. This situation violates good management practice as described by Shea (1960, p. 134), namely, that the organizational structure should arise from the job to be done and not be imposed from the top.

Hospital organization should be tailored to the client's care and needs. Some of the changes in the formal structure that are presently taking place include decentralizing authority; shortening the chains of command as the level of competency allows; widening the spans of control so that there is a flatter organizational structure; sharing responsibility and authority so that management can rely on expectation and accountability; and electing representative worker and consumer groups to participate in management decision making (Georgopoulos 1972, pp. 4–5).

An alternative to the traditional hierarchical pyramid structure is a matrix organization; this organization is structured according to a specific project or program, rather than to a function or department. In a matrix organization, the skills of specialists from different areas in the organization are utilized for a problem-centered, program-oriented approach. Matrix organizations are characterized by the teamwork of multidisciplinary specialists working on a specific task; the temporary nature of the task to be accomplished; and the fact that the tasks are extensions of and complements to the overall objectives of the organization (Anders 1975, p. 12). The use of matrix structures gives the organization flexibility to accomplish specific goals. Matrices are not replacements for traditional structures; they are merely superimposed on the usual structure in order to enable individuals to focus on a special project. The major disadvantage to a matrix structure is that it requires sophisticated management to mediate conflicting demands and loyalties between departmental and project affiliations (Schaefer 1976, p. 13). Examples of matrix organizations in hospitals include cardiopulmonary resuscitation teams, multidisciplinary client care teams, and research groups. In contrast to functional structuring, matrix organization emphasizes peer relationships, direct horizontal communication and authority chains, horizontal and diagonal work flows, management across functional and organizational lines, multilateral objectives, and a finite duration for the project (Longest 1976, p. 118).

The informal structure of the traditional hospital also places constraints on the workers' professional growth and maturity. A particular source of conflict is the doctor-nurse relationship. Kalisch and Kalisch (1977, pp. 51–55) cite many reasons for the poor communication between doctors and nurses, including a pattern of dominance by doctor and deference by nurse, doctors' devaluation of nursing, inadequate knowledge of the other profession, nursing's greater emphasis on psychosocial aspects, nurses' retreat from direct client care, the wider range of nursing education, two systems of authority, nurses' lack of career commitment, ambiguity of role functions, nurses' lack of control over nursing, doctors' fear of losing control, and political conflicts. Communication problems frustrate collaborative efforts to work together, emotionally exhaust the health care workers, prohibit satisfying social relationships, and reduce opportunities to provide expert care.

Solving the communication dilemma requires approaches at various system levels. The women's movement in the suprasystem is permeating the hospital organization to change attitudes toward nurses' roles in the organization as well as women's roles in society. Education and interdisciplinary knowledge can be used to socialize nurses and doctors to work collaboratively as team members. Nurses themselves are prepared to assume direct client care responsibilities as clinical specialists and nurse practitioners of primary care. Also, nurses are becoming more assertive in

initiating direct, nondefensive communication with doctors as professional and social equals. Communication strategies are being employed on
a one-to-one basis and within organized groups to change the stereotyped
image of nursing. As ideologies and personalities become more compatible, the health care received by the consumer will be enhanced by the
working relationships between nurses and doctors (Beyers and Phillips
1971, p. 5).

SUMMARY

An organization is an open social system in which groups of people combine knowledge, techniques, skills, and resources to accomplish a goal-
oriented task by integrating their structured activities. The organizational
environment is composed of interrelated subsystems, including the physical plant, the workers, the formal structure, the informal work groups, the
task, the management process, the organizational climate, and the style of
leadership. Organizations relate to their environments by either responsive or effective behaviors.

Organization management may take the form of the traditional, the
human relations, or the systems approach. The systems approach is believed to be the most comprehensive and useful because its emphasis is
not just task-oriented or people-oriented. The systems approach focuses
on the dynamic process of integrating and coordinating activities and interrelationships in a complex organizational system that is in continuous
interaction with its environment.

Organizational structure is the means by which an organization seeks
to achieve its objectives. Structure refers to the grouping of positions and
the establishment of patterns of relationships. Organizations have both a
formal and an informal structure. The formal structure is a deliberate plan
that emphasizes organizational positions in terms of authority and function. Authority, responsibility, accountability, organizational charts, decentralization, span of control, and line and staff positions are aspects of
the formal structure that affect nursing management. The informal structure pertains to the people and their relationships that arise spontaneously
as a result of working together. With advantages as well as disadvantages,
the informal structure gives life and flexibility to the formal organization.
Organizational structures vary according to the purpose, the people, the
task, and the work environment.

The organizational climate is the prevailing emotional atmosphere
that is shaped by the managers to reflect their values. Leadership styles
significantly influence the climate. Effective nurse-managers adapt their
leadership style to the work environment. Using a combination of autocratic and democratic behaviors according to the situation, nurse-managers

can facilitate the accomplishment of organizational objectives and the development of their subordinates' professional growth.

Hospital organizations are specialized sociotechnical systems composed of people who work to solve particular human problems. Hospitals are often handicapped by their bureaucratic-like structure. Decentralization, shared decision making, autonomous professionals, and matrix organization are alternatives that can modify the traditional multilevel, hierarchical structure. The informal structure can also be dysfunctional if doctors and nurses experience conflict and poor communication patterns. Efforts to collaborate as effective team members are improving as a result of the women's movement, education, the use of matrix organization, and the fact that nurses are becoming more assertive and direct in communicating as professional practitioners.

REFERENCES

Anders, Robert L. 1975. Matrix organization: an alternative for clinical specialists. *Journal of Nursing Administration* 7,6:11–14.

Arnold, Mary F. 1968. Professionalism and changing concepts of administration. *Journal of Nursing Education:* 7,5:10, 24–26.

Beyers, Marjorie and Phillips, Carole. 1971. *Nursing management for patient care.* Boston: Little, Brown.

Brief, Arthur P. 1976. Turnover among hospital nurses: a suggested model. *Journal of Nursing Administration* 6,10:55–57.

Bucklow, Maxine. 1973. A new role for the work group. In *Readings in managerial psychology,* ed. Harold J. Leavitt and Louis R. Pondy. Chicago: University of Chicago Press, pp. 458–475.

Claus, Karen E.; and Bailey, June T. 1977. *Power and influence in health care.* St. Louis: Mosby.

Davis, Keith. 1972. *Human behavior at work,* 4th ed. New York: McGraw-Hill.

Douglass, Laura Mae; and Bevis, Em Olivia. 1974. *Nursing leadership in action.* St. Louis: Mosby.

Dyer, William G. 1972. *The sensitive manipulator.* Provo, Utah: Brigham Young University Press.

Gaynor, Alan K.; and Berry, Rosalie K. 1973. Observations of a staff nurse: an organizational analysis. *Journal of Nursing Administration* 3,3:43–49.

Georgopoulos, Basil S., ed. 1972. *Organization research on health institutions.* Ann Arbor, Mich.: University of Michigan Press.

Heimann, Carol Grangaard. 1976. Four theories of leadership. *Journal of Nursing Administration* 6,6:18–24.

Hersey, Paul; Blanchard, Kenneth H.; and LaMonica, Elaine L. 1976. A situational approach to supervision. *Supervisor Nurse* 7,5:17–22.

Kalisch, Beatrice J.; and Kalisch, Philip A. 1977. An analysis of the sources of physician-nurse conflict. *Journal of Nursing Administration* 7,1:51–57.

Kast, Fremont E.; and Rosenzweig, James E. 1974. *Organization and management*, 2nd ed. New York: McGraw-Hill.

Levenstein, Aaron. 1976. The art and science of supervision: hospital climate. *Supervisor Nurse* 7,8:53–54.

Longest, Beaufort B., Jr. 1976. *Management practices for the health professional*. Reston, Va.: Reston Publishing.

Maccoby, Michael. 1976. *The gamesman*. New York: Simon and Schuster.

McGregor, Douglas. 1960. *The human side of enterprise*. New York: McGraw-Hill.

Mahowald, Jane; Freeman, John; and Dietsche, Bonnie. 1974. Decentralization of nursing authority. *Supervisor Nurse* 5,3:40–46.

Metcalfe, J. L. 1976. Organizational strategies and interorganizational networks. *Human Relations* 29,4:327–343.

O'Donovan, Thomas R. 1975. Leadership dynamics. *Journal of Nursing Administration* 5,9:32–35.

Price, Marjorie; Franck, Phyllis; and Veith, Shirley. 1974. *Nursing management: a programmed text*. New York: Springer.

Schaefer, Marguerite J. 1976. How should we organize? *Journal of Nursing Administration* 6,2:12–14.

————. 1975. Managing complexity. *Journal of Nursing Administration* 5,5:13–16.

Shea, Edmund. 1960. A hospital administrator says. . . . *Nursing Outlook* 8,3:134–140.

Simms, Laura L. 1973. Administration changes and implications for nursing practice in the hospital. *Nursing Clinics of North America* 8,2:227–234.

Smith, David. 1972. Organizational theory and the hospital. *Journal of Nursing Administration* 2,3:19–24.

Stevens, Barbara J. 1975. *The nurse as executive*. Wakefield, Mass.: Contemporary Publishing.

Stitely, Doris M. 1973. The role of the division head in a decentralized nursing service system. *Nursing Clinics of North America* 8,2: 247–255.

Chapter 3

Planning Considerations

Carolyn Chambers Clark

OBJECTIVES

After studying this chapter, the learner will:

- Define planning
- List questions to ask about objectives
- List questions to ask about a budget
- List ways to use time efficiently
- Identify staffing considerations
- List important interviewing considerations
- Identify ways to be an effective leader
- Describe ways to plan for change
- Identify several methods of handling conflict

DEFINITION OF THE PLANNING PROCESS

Plans are often identified as short-term or long-term. Short-term plans may later become long-term ones, since time factors may be less critical than the achievement of a desired outcome (Frey 1976). In order to be able to plan at the subsystem level, the nurse-manager must be aware of long-term plans at the system level.

The planning process in nursing begins with a philosophy of nursing, which should include what the nurse service is and what the expected outcomes from that service are. The nurse-manager plans in accordance with the current standards for nursing services as stated by the American Nurses Association. In addition, the nurse-manager must be knowledgeable about other subsystem, system, and suprasystem interfaces in the health care delivery system in order to prepare the organization for an ever changing future.

Planning comprises a number of interacting and overlapping processes. Planning can be defined according to the subskills needed to be an effective planner. Planning uses conceptualization skills, estimates of the number of physical resources, and inputs from personnel and consumer groups to form an integrated whole that can easily be communicated; is in line with institutional objectives, yet allows flexibility; is economically feasible and professionally sound; makes wise use of resources; and indicates how to put plans into action.

Since planning requires conceptualization skills, abstract ideas must be translated into specific decisions and actions. Planning is rarely finished because of the complex and ever changing physical and social systems with which the nurse-manager must work. To be effective, planning must be flexible, allowing for unforeseen circumstances. Although the head nurse or nursing supervisor may have decided on a staffing plan, unforeseen circumstances such as illness must be taken into account and an alternate plan must be worked out. Planning includes an ability to estimate the human and physical resource needs of a system. Current and past statistics that are pertinent to the system must be used in planning, such as the number and type of clients served and admitted; the percentage of various resources used; the types of referrals; the number, skill, and turnover of available personnel (Frey 1976).

Planning is not an individual activity. Formal decision making often requires on-the-spot answers. Effective planning includes input from consumer and professional groups; such groups can help the manager study facts and solve problems around critical issues (Frey 1976). If a satellite clinic in the community is being planned, it is necessary to secure suggestions and advice from appropriate personnel and consumers. Peters (1974) lists the following steps in the institutional planning process:

1 Convince the board.
2 Organize for planning.
3 Develop planning competence.
4 Take a hard look at the institution and what it does.

5 Organize a data-gathering procedure to learn about the consumer group and its health needs, and other providers of health services.
6 Adopt some guidelines for planning and operating the institution.
7 Determine long- and short-term institutional goals.
8 Set specific goals.
9 Establish priorities.
10 Identify alternative means to achieve goals.
11 Select a desired action or prepare a plan.
12 Decide on the means to carry out the action or plan.
13 Obtain approval for action or plan.
14 Carry out the action or plan.
15 Evaluate.

Let the community participate as much as possible in every step of the process.

CHOOSING OBJECTIVES

To be an effective manager, the nurse must have analyzed the organizational environment and its constraints. Having enough information about what is and what is possible, the manager can eliminate unreasonable risk and plan for success. Objectives are often specified in terms of method or process, for example, "Referrals will be made as needed." When objectives are listed in this way rather than in terms of the desired results, there is the risk that interventions will be continued even though they have already achieved the objective (Cantor 1976, p. 9). Behavioral objectives specify the expected outcomes and are precise enough so that it is clear whether or not they have been attained. Behavioral objectives use action verbs and delineate specific behaviors (Mager 1962). Objectives should specify what is to be done when.

Managers frequently become caught up in the daily, immediate problems, and give little attention to long-range plans or prevention (Matsunaga 1975). Sherwin (1976) explains this as a conflict between maintenance and change objectives, and suggests that project teams should be given authority and responsibility to effect one or more change objectives. Whether Sherwin's suggestion is used or not, there should be a balance between maintenance and change objectives. The following are questions that the nurse-manager can ask to determine if the objectives are effective:

1 Are the objectives based on sound analysis (as opposed to hunches)?
2 Are there objectives to cover all important phases of the system's operation?
3 Are the objectives clear and specific?

4   Are the objectives consistent with the framework of the organization?

5   Are the objectives expressed in quantifiable terms?

6   Are the objectives attainable within a specified time period?

7   Are the objectives high enough, yet attainable?

8   Are the objectives weighted in terms of priority?

9   Is there a balance between long- and short-term objectives?

10   Are the objectives available in writing?

11   If each nurse-manager were asked to write his or her understanding of the subsystem's objectives, would there be a high degree of agreement?

12   Are the objectives future oriented?

13   Are the objectives used as a guide for daily decision making?

14   Are the objectives meaningful to those who must meet them?

15   Are there enough objectives to provide direction, yet not so many that the people affected are not overwhelmed?

16   Are there objectives that provide for both maintenance and change within the system?

Management by objectives (MBO) is a business term that is defined differently by different authors. Kast and Rosenzweig (1974, p. 171) discuss MBO as an attempt to include all levels of management in the process of setting goals. In this view, the manager works with his or her personnel to establish specific goals and the plans for achieving those goals. This approach seems quite simple, but there are pitfalls. First, enough time must be allowed to receive feedback, modify objectives, and evaluate feedback about the modification. Second, a major issue in this approach is whether the objectives should be established at the top and then communicated to the workers, or whether lower-level personnel should participate in setting their own objectives. Probably systems that are bureaucratic in structure establish objectives at the top, provide little communication, and allow little input from below. Management by objectives is most successful when collaboration, cooperation, and team efforts are encouraged. Third, MBO often focuses primarily on tasks (Beer and Ruh 1976) and tends to maintain dynamic equilibrium; recognizing the desired outcome for a task such as cleaning equipment may be relatively easy, but recognizing the desired outcome for increasing preventive health behavior is more difficult. Fourth, MBO does not help managers to evaluate what went wrong (or right) in the objective-attainment process; MBO merely gives information about whether a result was attained or not.

Given these drawbacks, MBO is successful because it allows the manager to judge results, not personalities, and because it tends to improve the quantity and quality of communication between the manager and other personnel or clients (Beer and Ruh 1976, p. 59). Strauss and Sayles (1972) stress the importance of MBO in providing feedback, motivating personnel, and encouraging independence.

MBO requires that the organizational objectives be integrated with personal needs and goals. It can be assumed that everyone has basic needs such as for rest, activity, food, and fluid, as well as other needs such as for recognition, self-esteem, and self-actualization. The manager would have to determine which of these needs has priority for a given individual. The organizational objectives and constraints would also be part of the knowledge base of the manager. Ganong and Ganong (1974, p. 22) describe the use of this approach at the two-person management level where a supervisor was able to motivate an L.P.N. to be on time for work by mutually setting a client goal, setting a date for its completion, and evaluating the results.

Henry (1975) describes a systems approach in which objectives fit within the total systems analysis. The procedure for using this approach includes:

1 Defining the system (or subsystem) to be investigated.
2 Defining the output as well as the means to measure the output.
3 Quantifying the elements of the system and quantifying their relationships. (In the case of preventive health visits, the elements might be: What is the effect of previous visits on the clients' level of knowledge; of the availability of health care workers; and of the cost of visits?).
4 Determining the desired measurable performance or output. (To achieve the objectives for preventive health visits, one must assess the physical plant, manager, health care worker, and client or family transportation system).
5 Determining the cost effectiveness of alternative methods to improve the system output. (For each dollar or energy unit, how many dollars' worth of improvement will be obtained in the total system?).
6 Implementing the most desirable decisions and measuring the results.

From examining the systems-analysis procedure, it is clear that objectives fit into the total process of management. They may need to be refined at several points in the planning or management process.

BUDGETING

Nurses are notoriously poor in money matters. Their pleas for health care are often based on ethical or moral issues rather than cost-benefit ratios (Stevens 1975). They may not have enough education or knowledge in this area. Although not every nurse will have to develop a budget, nurses are often asked to provide information for budgets and so they need to know the components and theory of budget-making. It is especially important for nurses to realize that money from one budget item cannot be frivolously transferred to another item without it having ramifications for the whole budget as well as the health care system within which the budget operates.

A budget can be thought of as one way to translate objectives into action (Stevens 1975). The budget can also be thought of as a plan for the future, a communication, and a control mechanism. One way to evaluate the performance of a head nurse or supervisor is in terms of his or her ability to achieve results specified within the cost constraints of the budget (Caplan 1971, p. 84).

Participative budgeting means that those who are responsible for performance under a budget participate in the budget-making decisions. Participative budgeting may have dysfunctional consequences for the organization for the following reasons: (1) Managers may underestimate revenues and overestimate costs in order to produce slack in their budgets, (2) There may be pseudoparticipation where decisions are made by top level administrators under the guise of wanting input from all who will be affected, (3) Lower performance standards may be set if budgeted objectives are accepted as personal objectives (Caplan 1971, pp. 86–87). Participative budgeting is most effective when there is frequent feedback and actual (not pseudo) participation.

Planning-programming-budgeting systems (PPBS) use a systems model. This is similiar to long-term planning approaches. The budget becomes the financial expression of the underlying program plan, and decisions are translated into requests for monies. PPBS focus on program output (specified objectives) whereas traditional budgetary approaches emphasize inputs. The total costs and benefits of various alternatives are assessed in an attempt to determine the rate of return for various programs. The organizational structure of the health care system and of hospital organizations is not often mission- or objective-oriented; rather, different systems or subsystems have similar or overlapping functions. PPBS develop subsystem elements that contribute to program accomplishment. Cost-benefit analysis is a specific application of systems analysis; it is an attempt to compare the costs of the alternate ways to attain a specific objective. For example, using a systems analysis approach in nursing care, it may be possible to compare the cost and benefits of community care for a group of clients versus inhospital treatment of a similar group, or of individual clinic health teaching programs versus group teaching programs. Such analyses are simple when used with a relatively closed system. They become exceedingly complex when economic, social, and human factors need to be evaluated. A program budget reallocates efforts from a yearly budget to long-term budgetary measures. Expenditures would be directly tied to program objectives. The budget would emphasize future needs rather than control of expenditures. The annual routine of preparing a budget would be converted into an appraisal and formulation of future programs. This would require a shift in informational input; essential information would be collected during the planning process and made available in usable form for the budgetary process. In this model, the program budget would cover at least a 5-year period (Johnson, Kast, and Rosenzweig 1973, pp. 426–440).

Some of the problems inherent in developing PPBS include the traditional emphasis of budgetary systems upon short-term, financial controls; the difficulty in developing a budget based on programs; and the difficulties that arise in the interface between various subsystems and systems (Johnson, Kast, and Rosenzweig 1973, pp. 449–450).

Hospital administrators may resist PPBS for the same reasons that Congress resists its development by governmental agencies—PPBS present a threat to the power and control of administrators. However, there is a trend to reimburse hospitals for actual services based on diagnosis, rather than on a per diem average cost of service (*New York Times,* March 6, 1977; February 27, 1977).

Participative budgeting and PPBS are trends of the future and they may not be found in the system in which the nurse-manager functions. That system may still be using a budgetary method where inputs are emphasized. Housley (1976) suggests that the supervisor examine the following budget components: personnel, supplies, capital equipment and improvement, and travel and education. Nurse-managers may need to consider the following when planning or examining a budget:

1   What has been the budget for the past year?
2   What is the projected salary increase?
3   What new programs are being contemplated, and what physical and human resources will be required?
4   Is there a projected increase or decrease in physical facilities such as beds, supplies, and operating rooms?
5   What is the projected percentage of occupancy or use of available resources?
6   Is there an organizational chart that can help to ensure that no personnel positions are overlooked in planning?
7   Do job descriptions for new personnel need to be written?
8   How is overtime computed and how should it be budgeted?
9   Can personnel positions be exchanged for one another? For example, can two aide positions be budgeted to make one R.N. position?)
10   Has there been a change in the general complexity of client care?
11   Has there been a functional change in job descriptions?

12   Will there be a change in educational programs necessitating an increased or decreased number of students, a time release for classroom hours, new educational media, a change in student/faculty ratios?

13   What additional personnel hours need to be budgeted to allow for vacations, illness, and educational needs?

14   How are fringe benefits calculated?

15   Are there costs for recruitment, orientation, and overlap of new and terminating personnel?

16   When does the organization consider new purchases as capital, rather than as operational expenditures?

17   What influence might a new technology or methodology have?

18   What coordination is there between nursing and medicine? (For example, do requests for medicine come out of the nursing budget?)

19   What changes in physician or nursing modes of therapy might affect the budget?

20   What changes in other systems or subsystems might affect nursing?

21   How is the cost of depreciation handled in the organization?

22   Which repair and renovation costs are handled within the organization and which are done by outside organizations?

23   How are indirect or overhead costs such as physical plant maintenance, heating, light, telephone, rental space, housekeeping, and general administration handled?

24   Are there hidden costs such as the servicing of gift equipment or the training of volunteers?

25   What is the rate of inflation for supplies or equipment?

26   What calculations need to be included to demonstrate that a new procedure, kind of supply, or equipment may save nursing hours?

27   What anticipated income is there from continuing education programs?

28   How can the income from nursing services be calculated?

29   What priority can be attached to each budget item?

30   How can supplies be ordered by a yearly amount to ensure a more accurate projection of the supply budget?

31   How can the supply budget be projected for each month?

32   Can quotations from at least three different manufacturers be secured in order to decide which piece of equipment to purchase?

33   How can outputs such as purchases and nursing services be quantified?

34   How much should be alloted for the travel and educational needs of personnel?

35   Is there a percentage (for example, 1 percent of the total budget) that should be budgeted for miscellaneous needs that may arise?

36   What record-keeping procedures will be needed to assure accountability?

37   How often should the budget-maker do a self-audit to guard against errors in projected costs or record-keeping?

38 What items in last year's budget will not need to be included this year?

USING TIME

The nurse-manager can use a combination of structuring the work day and delegating tasks and responsibilities in order to use time most constructively. Specific times can be scheduled for doing certain tasks. Uninterrupted planning time should be allowed for. This time is used to set priorities and anticipate problems for a given day so that potential crises can be handled most effectively.

Office practices, operating style, and standard operating procedures should be decided on and communicated clearly to coworkers. For example, others should not be allowed to interrupt the manager's planning time unless there is a crisis; conferences and telephone conversations should be to the point; agendas and written memos can be used to emphasize what issues will be covered in upcoming meetings; newly admitted clients are to have a nursing history taken according to a prescribed guide. The manager should not accept coworkers' responsibilities. The manager may help the other person to solve problems around the issue, but it is not the manager's job to do the task.

The manager needs to develop a system for undertaking unpleasant tasks. It is important to set up an easy feedback system for all plans. When several people need to be informed about an issue or task, an agenda can be sent, and a group meeting can be held to inform everyone about the matter at once and to have an opportunity for feedback (Comte and Lee 1975, pp. 19–21).

When delegating a task, it is important to state clearly, preferably in writing, just what the job entails. What may be obvious to the manager may be new to the person who must undertake the task. Time should be taken to review the task with the coworker; more will be accomplished if the other person understands clearly what is expected and what standards can be used to determine when the task has been completed. The manager will have to evaluate which persons need to have everything spelled out in detail. Some people require repetition and feedback before they can begin a task or complete it adequately. Whenever a job is delegated, the manager must check to see that it has been completed; this does not mean snooping or badgering the other, but does mean some kind of periodic assessment of the task or goal attainment. This might include frequent observation, informal or formal meetings, and written reports. Whenever a job is delegated, it is the manager's responsibility to ask how the other feels about doing it. It is wise to separate two issues: whether a certain task is going to be delegated or not, and how the other feels about being given the task. Some workers may have low self-esteem and feel that they cannot take on more; they may need to be helped to become more independent by being told of their progress and by being assigned responsibility in small areas. It may help if the manager smooths the way by telling them what areas of responsibility have been delegated so that they will be prepared for the change.

It is important to keep the person to whom responsibility is being delegated informed of any new plans and problems that may affect his or her managing. Giving responsibility means giving authority. An assistant will probably not do the task in the same way the manager would; as long as results are forthcoming, the manager should not interfere. When mistakes occur, the manager should discuss it in private; when results are achieved, workers should be praised in public (Pollock 1971).

STAFFING

In theory, staffing is an attempt to translate objectives into the kind of care the organization wishes to provide. In practice, both scientific methods and intuitive experience approaches have flaws. A major proponent of the scientific method of staffing lists the following eleven steps to take (Ramey 1973):

1   Obtain a representative survey of each client unit to determine the number of clients requiring intensive, moderate, and minimal care.

2   Develop a client data-collection form listing direct and indirect nursing activities.

3   Survey each specialty unit separately.

4   Designate two or three nurses to collect data for 24 hours on each client on each selected unit.

5   Establish the number of minutes needed to accomplish each nursing activity safely.

6   Specify the amount of time needed for new functions such as assessment, planning, teaching, counseling, and evaluation.

7   Designate which activities should be performed by professional nurses or auxiliary personnel.

8   Determine how many staff members are required on duty on a daily basis

$$\left(\frac{\text{hours of care/client} \times \text{number of clients}}{\text{hours worked/employee}} \right)$$

9   Obtain the number of client days/year/client unit.

10   Calculate the total number of nursing hours/year/unit (taking into account holidays, vacations, and so forth).

11   Allow hours for inservice education, administration of the unit, orientation of new staff, and participation in community and research projects.

In addition to this method of staffing, Aydelotte (1973) discusses the industrial engineering, management engineering, and operation research methods. E. Clark (1977) suggests that staffing patterns should be based on a direct analysis of client needs rather than on a description of what nurses do for patients. Scientific methods of staffing require extensive research to develop a data base for decision making.

Stevens (1975) points out that a system is ever changing and should be flexible where staffing is concerned. She suggests a number of contingency plans to provide for system changes. One plan is the internal transfer of staff from one unit to another. However, a disadvantage of this plan is that the unity of the work group is threatened, and the transferred worker is often resentful. A variation of this plan is to use a "float staff," composed of workers who like the challenge of ever changing work and settings. In either of these plans, the nurse-manager needs to develop a reward system that will recognize the disadvantages of constant changes at work. To develop such a system, the manager must understand what is rewarding to staff members.

Some of the rewards that nurses say will decrease their dissatisfaction are: more educational programs; reimbursement for taking courses; recognition for performing well; a salary increase, more vacation days, and two more weekends off per month; working a straight day shift; being able to work part time; being given more responsibility; opportunities to do nursing research; assistance in improving job skills; having a different supervisor; and advancing in one's career (McCloskey 1975).

Different levels of workers may find different rewards in work. For example, it may be important to eighth-grade graduates to feel that they are doing a good job and are cooperative, to have a supervisor who seeks their opinions without being excessively critical, to receive higher pay, and to have a chance to use their skills. High school graduates are more likely to want to learn more skills, to have the opportunity to work through conflict, to be able to use their skills, to be asked for their opinions, and to feel a sense of accomplishment. College graduates seem to want to have a more active role in decision-making and authority, to be respected and accepted by others, and to obtain assistance from coworkers (Carey et al. 1976).

In addition to understanding what is rewarding to the average staff member, the nurse-manager can ask staff members which of the following needs is most important to them: economic, dominance over others, recognition, security and reassurance, or belonging (Kafka 1973). Using the above information, the nurse-manager can devise ways to reward and motivate a "float staff."

A second plan mentioned by Stevens (1975, p. 134) is a reserve pool of part-time workers. Under this arrangement, a regular group of nurses such as young mothers or housewives agree to work on call when the need arises. Some institutions rotate oncall hours among regular personnel. However, oncall systems are costly because nurses often receive a base oncall pay whether they are needed for work or not. Oncall and overtime work is also costly because it exerts a psychological and physiological drain on the affected staff.

A companion floor system allows for two floors to serve as relief for one another. Personnel from both floors can be oriented to their companion floor before being transferred. This system would decrease the stress of unfamiliarily that occurs when workers have to adapt to a new setting and new people frequently.

An alternative plan is to move clients. Under this plan, clients are assigned to units according to their anticipated care needs at the time of their admission. This arrangement requires that several units be available, that admission information be sufficient for assignment, that information about the status of each unit be available, and that the admission nurse have the authority and knowledge to make placement decisions (Stevens 1975, p. 135).

Changes in the workload within the work day create staffing problems. Ways to decrease the flux include distributing bathing activities over shifts, bargaining for staggered visiting hours by physicians, and increasing the number of self-directed, professional nurses.

The seven-day work week creates problems in planning for full-time nurses because planned work days per year cannot be equally divided. Ways to handle this problem include using overstaffed days for inservice education, transferring one nurse to an overloaded unit, and hiring nurses who will work four days a week. Vacation schedules, illness, and personal requests compound the problem of staffing. Central staffing, rules for handling requests for exceptions, and computerized staffing can alleviate these problems.

Staffing needs are also affected by the type of assignment system used. One type, the functional, divides labor into a treatment nurse, bedside nurse, medication nurse, and so on. This system requires minimal time for coordination. Although the interpersonal needs of workers and clients may be overlooked in this system, it is efficient and often used in times of staff shortage. Under this system, the head nurse is the manager and performs most management functions. Since many different nurses are likely to see the client, errors or health care omissions will probably be caught.

The team method requires more of the head nurse's coordinating, observational, management, teaching, and evaluation time. Responsibility is delegated from the head nurse to team leaders. With the unit divided into two or more teams, the nurse has responsibility for fewer clients; in theory, more time can be spent on care and there can be a better match between staff abilities and client needs. Using this method, there may be more errors because the worker does multiple, different tasks. Thus, more time is spent monitoring for errors. Some studies have shown that team nursing has hidden costs such as requiring a minimum of six team leaders to plan and coordinate nursing care for a seven-day period. With so many managers, it may not be clear who is responsible for continuity of care (E. Clark, 1977).

Modular nursing is the assignment of a small module of clients to a nurse. Efficiency may be lost since staff mobility is reduced; however, there are fewer organizational tasks. Closer monitoring of care may reduce care errors and increase the likelihood of meeting client needs (Stevens 1975, pp. 140–141).

Primary care is the assignment of a client to one nurse throughout the care process. The focus here is primarily on planning rather than on implementing the plan. Consistency of care is increased because one nurse plans for the 24-hour care of a client. In theory, the nurse should feel more satisfied with this system because the work results are visible. Nurses must be confident and skilled professionals to be able to work effectively under this plan. From functional to primary care nursing, the head nurse's role has changed from that of organizer and manager of tasks to evaluator of care and teacher of nurses (Stevens 1975, pp. 141–143).

INTERVIEWING

The nurse-manager must have a firm grasp of interviewing and communication skills. During their education, nurses have usually had practice in the nondirective style of communicating with clients, and sometimes in using a structured interview form or guide to do nursing histories. The nurse-manager may be participating in decision-making, problem-solving, or information-exchange interviews. Examples of such interviews include the selection of personnel, handling of unsolved client care problems, and termination interviews. No matter what the type of interview, the nurse-manager can benefit from the following guidelines (Pollock 1971; Dunn 1972; Strauss 1972):

1   Allow ample time for the interview.
2   Become familiar with the employee facts (and omissions) by studying job applications, written requests, and other available data before the interview.
3   Devise a list of questions or areas to be covered; refer to it during the interview.
4   Conduct the interview in a private area.

5 Allow no interruptions or unnecessary digressions.

6 Avoid asking questions that can be answered with a "yes" or "no."

7 Listen to what the interviewee says; do not assume you know what will be said.

8 Observe the interviewee's nonverbal communication; it may provide clues.

9 Do not ask questions that have already been answered in written form; use the interview to fill in gaps and obtain details.

10 Record information during the interview because one's recall diminishes rapidly.

11 Answers that appear too general should be made more precise, for example, "Give an example of that," or "Tell me what you mean by. . . ."

12 Answers that are too wordy or off the point should be refocused, for example, "Before you go on, tell me more about . . .," or "I think I understand the problem; let's go on to. . . ."

13 If interviewing more than one person about the same issue, cover exactly the same topics with all of them; this will provide more consistent, valid information.

14 Avoid putting the other "on-the-spot"; ask a less threatening question if you notice the interviewee is becoming more anxious.

15 Be sure you do less than half of the talking; encourage the interviewee to comment with statements such as, "Go on," "Tell me what has happened," and "What are your ideas?"

16 Help the interviewee think through the problem with comments such as, "What do you think the effect of that would be?" "What solutions have you tried?" "How have you tried to handle that?"

17 Avoid discussing irrelevant topics.

18 Avoid jumping to conclusions without sufficient information.

19 Avoid trying to guess what the interviewee thinks, feels, or means; ask him or her.

20 Avoid arguing; when you disagree, use comments such as, "That's one way to look at it," or "I disagree, but I see your point."

21 Avoid stating what the interviewee's motives for action are; this leads to defensiveness and amateur psychotherapy.

22 Avoid giving advice until all the facts are known and the interviewee has been encouraged to come to his or her own conclusions.

23 Repeat complex directions several times and then ask for feedback from the interviewee to make sure that the directions were understood.

24 Avoid putting words in the interviewee's mouth with comments such as, "Don't you think it would be best if. . . ?"

25 Avoid making snap decisions to hire, fire, or grant a request based on your feeling in the interview; when making important decisions, weigh the pros and cons carefully outside of the interview; tell the interviewee that you will get back to him or her when you have thought through the alternatives.

26 Remember to keep charge of the interview by beginning, guiding, and ending it.

27 Summarize what has been accomplished at the end of the interview.

28 State what specific action will follow from the interview, for example, "I will share this information with Mr. Jones and I will let you know if your request has been granted next Tuesday morning."

LEADING

All leaders motivate others to achieve desired goals (Tannenbaum, Weschler, and Massarik 1974). Leadership used to be thought of as a quality, but now leadership is viewed as a set of functions that need to be filled (C. Clark 1977). The nurse-manager, as designated leader, may fulfill only some of these functions; others may be encouraged or taught to fill other functions. Leadership functions include both task and maintenance functions. Task functions are those that are related directly to the accomplishment of organizational or group objectives. The following behaviors are task-oriented:

1 Initiating the task by saying, for example, "Let's begin the meeting."

2 Keeping others working on the task, for example, "How can we cut down on the time it takes to prepare the unit?" or "In our last meeting, we decided to work on objective 1; let's get to that now."

3 Clarifying unclear statements or behaviors, for example, "I'm not sure I understand your request; what is it?" or "Who are you talking about?"

4 Suggesting ways to solve the problem or achieve the goal, for example, "Let's try pooling ideas on this," or "I suggest we try Rena's solution."

5 Pointing out movement toward (or away from) the goal, for example, "We're off the topic," or "You requested an answer today and I haven't given it to you yet."

6 Restating or summarizing, for example, "If I heard you correctly. . . ." or "So far we've covered. . . ."

7 Refocusing on the task, for example, "Before we go into that, let's finish this," or "Go back and finish Ms. Johnson's care."

8 Giving information and setting deadlines, for example, "Your report is due Thursday at 2 P.M." or "I'll let you know the answer to your question tomorrow at 1 P.M."

Maintenance functions pertain to the improvement of interpersonal work relationships. The following behaviors are maintenance-oriented:

1 Giving recognition and support, for example, "You did a fine job today," or "You seem upset; let's go into my office and discuss it."

2 Relieving tension, for example, "Let's sit on this 'til tomorrow" or using a sense of humor.

3 Encouraging directness, for example, "I can't answer for Ms. Thompkins—ask her directly," or "I'd like to talk with you about this problem."

4 Voicing implied feeling, for example, "I sense these changes are creating problems," or "I wonder if you're frustrated with your assignment."

5 Encouraging evaluation, for example, "I've told you how I see your work; now you evaluate it," or "How do you think we're doing on this?"

6 Agreeing or accepting, for example, "That's a good idea," or "I see your point."

7 Keeping communication open, for example, setting up meetings where staff members are encouraged to share ideas, arranging "open hours" when employees can drop by to discuss work-related problems, or establishing a suggestion box to receive feedback from employees.

Appropriate leadership must adapt to an ever changing system. Not all decisions require input from the group; if that were the case, there would be little, if any, action. In situations where the employee group does not have adequate skills or time, or is experiencing a crisis, the manager should make decisions, structure tasks by directing others' behavior, and attempt to reduce tension. In situations where the employee group has adequate skills, time, interest, and comfort, the manager should share responsibility and leadership functions. By teaching others to lead, the manager makes sure that the system can function without his or her presence. Managers who have strong needs to control others and situations will find it difficult to share responsibility and leadership functions.

The nurse-manager who wants to be an effective leader can increase cohesiveness within the work group and serve as an advocate to the system or suprasystem. Cohesiveness is a measure of the group's attractiveness to its members. The manager can increase the attractiveness of the work group by making it better serve the needs of the members. A group will be more attractive if it encourages cooperation, permits free discussion, and recognizes its members' accomplishments (Cartwright and Zander 1953, p. 82).

Groups that have a high level of cohesiveness influence their members to achieve group goals and meet interpersonal needs. The leader can increase cohesiveness by making sure that the goals are relevant and clearly stated, that cooperation among the members is promoted, and that paths to achievement are clear and rewarded when attained. Cohesiveness is also increased when the group members are asked for their opinion, when there is frequent cooperative interaction, when the similarities among the group members are highlighted, when activities are planned to increase the potential for attaining success, and when feelings can be expressed (C. Clark 1977).

Being able to serve as an advocate for the group means that the manager must be able to articulate clearly and convincingly the group's concerns. This presupposes open communication and trust between the manager and managed, as well as enthusiasm for and an ability to project the group's needs and wishes. If the nurse-manager can foster cooperation and trust among the work group, yet cannot negotiate for reasonable work conditions, this is not effective leadership. The nurse-manager might consider the following questions to determine the effectiveness of his or her leadership:

1 Are both task and maintenance functions being fulfilled?
2 Does leadership vary depending upon the system variables?
3 Is leadership being shared?
4 Is work group cohesiveness being promoted?
5 Are the work group's concerns being clearly articulated to other relevant systems or suprasystems?

PLANNING FOR CHANGE

The nurse-manager may be most successful in planning for change by viewing the organization as an adaptive, problem-solving system that operates in a complicated, rapidly changing environment (Bennis 1966, p. 47). Despite the manager's view, resistance to change is quite likely in all organizations, but especially in bureaucracies. In a bureaucratic organization one often finds that: conflict is suppressed; resources are centrally controlled; rewards of money, power, and status are more available than satisfaction in one's work; workers have no right to appeal decisions; a conservation orientation prevails where change is perceived as threatening; feelings of anxiety and chronic dissatisfaction pervade the environment; the organization is staffed primarily by nonprofessionals; and it is understood (if not made explicit) that failure is not allowed (Davis 1971, p. 253).

Whether organizations are bureaucratic or not, there will be a resistance to change when the nature of the change is not made clear to the workers; when different people see different meanings in the proposed change; when there are strong forces to change and not to change; when persons affected by the change have pressure put on them to change, yet have no voice in the nature or direction of the change; when the change is made because of personal factors rather than because of impersonal requirements or sanctions; and when the change ignores already established institutions in the group (Davis 1971, p. 265).

Organizations change in their own right, but if a manager chooses to introduce change, the following questions must be addressed: What is to be accomplished? Why? What are the advantages and disadvantages of introducing the change? What methods will be used to implement the change? In answering these questions, the manager should consider how the change will affect work habits, how people relate to and regard their work, and what the established relationships are among workers and with the organization.

Certain principles that have been derived from research on change help the nurse-manager. Two types of individuals can be identified in relation to change: early adopters and late adopters. Early adopters tend to be younger, have a higher social status, be less dogmatic, have more formal education, and be able to deal well with abstractions (Davis 1971, p. 232). These characteristics are more likely to be associated with the baccalaureate-educated, professional nurse, as opposed to the nonprofessional health worker. Both early and late adopters will accept change more readily if they have participated in the preliminary planning and decision making (Davis 1971, p. 224).

There are three means by which the nurse-manager can communicate information about an upcoming change: by interpersonal or face-to-face contact, by using mass media channels, and by arranging forums where small groups discuss a mass media program. According to the purpose of the communication, different channels or combinations should be selected. For example, mass media channels are preferable for early adopters, and when awareness of ideas, innovation, and decision-making input are required; interpersonal channels are preferable for late adopters and for those who value group membership, as well as for persuasion and changing attitudes. Despite the channel, communication about change is most likely to be accepted if the source is credible and not viewed as antagonistic. The emotional impact of "bad news" can be reduced if workers are told in advance that there will be bad news. Messages about change are most likely to be accepted if little anxiety is aroused, if the major arguments for changing are presented at the outset, if the message can be communicated through more than one of the senses, is consistent with existing knowledge and attitudes, and is receiver- rather than source-oriented. A period of stress or crisis seems to produce rumors that spread through the informal, interpersonal channels, as well as more rapid adoption of an innovation (Davis 1971, pp. 223–231).

The nurse-manager can initiate change in a number of ways. First, he or she can decide on the change; communicate clearly what is to be done, by whom, when, and in what way; and then follow up to make sure that the change has occurred. Another method is to employ an independent change agent to serve as a catalyst in the change process. Or, a design group or working committee may be charged with the responsibility for participating in decision making or implementing the change. Another method is to arrange for staff members to evaluate the change over a trial period. Once they have responsibility for the new behaviors, their attitudes toward the change may become more positive. Despite careful planning, there may be unanticipated outcomes since it is not always possible to predict the system effects of change. Using the information presented here, the nurse-manager may want to devise a planning list whenever change is to be introduced; the following points might be considered:

1   Is the organization bureaucratic?
2   What forces are facilitating or hindering change?
3   What input do those who will be affected by the change have?
4   What established group institutions may be affected by the change?
5   What work habits will be altered by the change?
6   What work and social relationships will be affected by the change?
7   How can early and late adopters be identified?
8   What channels of communication would be most effective in promoting the change?
9   How can the message about change be presented so it will be received most favorably?
10   Is a period of stress or crisis likely to affect the adoption of the change?
11   How will the effects of the change be evaluated?

HANDLING CONFLICT

Conflict occurs when opposing viewpoints, forces, or issues confront individuals, groups, or organizations (Veninga 1974, p. 13). Conflict can be either constructive or destructive; it can lead to curiosity, struggle, and growth, or it can lead to decreased efficiency and an inability to meet objectives if the opposing forces are not brought into the open. Nurse-managers must be knowledgeable about conflict and its resolution.

The first step in handling conflict is to assess the sources of conflict; some of the sources include: assigning an impossible task, not defining a task clearly, jockeying for power or status, having loyalties to outside groups, working hard at the task. Depending upon the assessment, the nurse-manager might decide to reassign duties, redefine a task, make provisions for interpersonal satisfaction and comfort, develop or emphasize shared loyalties within the group, or accept the fact that some disagreement may be useful to task accomplishment.

Several interventions have traditionally been used in organizations that may be useful in the short range: avoiding conflict, smoothing over or minimizing differences, and compelling others to accept authoritarian decisions. More useful conflict-resolution methods include: bargaining or compromise, confronting the problem; mutual alliances or common pacts, altering the resources or structures, and working committees. Labor-management arbitration is an example of bargaining or compromise. It requires that each party give up something, and that each party recognize the other's claims. The outcome depends upon the balance of power between the two parties (Lewis 1976, pp. 18–22).

Confrontation can occur on a one-to-one basis or within or between groups. Here, the problem is mutually defined. Each party delineates the areas of difference or controversy and then attempts to have an objective discussion of them. Veninga (1974) has mentioned specific ways the nurse-manager can use confrontation with an employee. The first step is to determine an appropriate time to attempt reconciliation. Next, the meeting should be held on neutral ground—in an undisturbed area where there will be enough time for the interview. Statements should be used that decrease defensiveness such as, "We are both responsible," "I want to work this out with you," or "How can we make sure that this problem won't occur again?"

Veninga (1974) warns that in a confrontation interview employees may be afraid that their jobs are in jeopardy, that they will be ostracized from the team, or that they will lose face or respect. To guard against these fears, the nurse-manager can convey that the two parties can disagree and still work together. The manager also needs to follow through on what was agreed upon in the interview.

Mutual alliance or common pact is a method whereby several groups in conflict come together to discuss their different interests. A series of meetings is arranged to negotiate a step-by-step resolution of differences. Various groups may align and realign themselves during the course of the meetings. Since group alliances will be based on interest and respect, new rules for relating can be developed (Leininger 1974).

T-groups (sensitivity training groups) can also be used to change behavior patterns. If the source of conflict is material resources, a way can probably be found to transfer energy or other resources for materials. Structural patterns of conflict can be changed by transferring certain group members to other responsibilities or projects or developing new work positions or grievance procedures. (Lewis 1976).

Supraordinate goals can be developed that require conflicting groups to work together for their mutual benefit. Working committees can be used to clarify goals and communication, as well as to increase work satisfaction.

SUMMARY

Planning comprises a number of interacting and overlapping processes. It uses conceptualization skills, estimates of the number of physical resources, and inputs from personnel and consumer groups. Planning is consistent with institutional objectives, yet allows flexibility; is economically feasible and professionally sound; makes wise use of resources; and indicates how to put plans into action. One step in the planning process is the development of specific short- and long-term objectives. Although not all nurses make budgets, they need to know how to plan and evaluate a budget. An important aspect of the planning process is the use of time; structuring the work day and delegating tasks and responsibilities can help the nurse-manager use time effectively. Staffing is an attempt to translate objectives into the kind of care the organization wishes to provide. There are several methods of staffing, including descriptive, industrial engineering, management engineering, operations research, and contingency planning. Staffing is also affected by the type of nurse-to-client assignment system that is used. Interviewing is a skill the nurse-manager must use to make decisions, solve problems, or exchange information.

The nurse-manager may be most effective as a leader if he or she can share leadership functions with others, promote work group cohesiveness, and articulate the group's concerns to other systems or subsystems convincingly. When planning for change in the organization, the nurse-manager should consider whether the organization is bureaucratic; what forces are acting to increase and decrease change; what input is important from those who will be affected by the change; what institutions, work habits, work and social relationships will be affected by the change; how to identify early and late adopters; what channels of communication will be most effective in promoting the change; how to present the message about change most effectively; how the change will be perceived; and how the effects of the change will be evaluated. When planning how to handle conflict, the nurse-manager should first assess the conflict. Next, the choice should be made among bargaining or compromise, confronting the problem, mutual alliances or common pacts, altering the resources or structures, and working committees.

REFERENCES

Aydelotte, Myrtle K. 1973. Staffing for high-quality care. *Nursing Digest* 1,7:72–75.

Beer, Michael; and Ruh, Robert A. 1976. Employee growth through performance management. *Harvard Business Review* 54,5:59–66.

Bennis, Warren. 1966. *Beyond bureaucracy: essays on the development of human organization.* New York: McGraw-Hill.

Cantor, Marjorie M. 1976. Philosophy, purpose, and objectives: why do we have them? In *Management for nurses: a multidisciplinary approach,* ed. Sandra Stone et al. St. Louis: Mosby, pp. 5–12.

Caplan, Edwin H. 1971. *Management accounting and behavioral science.* Reading, Mass.: Addison-Wesley.

Carey, Raymond G; Johnson, Homer; and Kerman, Fred. 1976. Improvement in employee morale linked to variety of agents. *Hospitals, J.A.H.A.* 50,18:85–87 and 90.

Cartwright, Dorwin; and Zander, Alvin. 1953. *Group dynamics: research and theory.* Evanston, Ill.: Row, Peterson.

Clark, Carolyn Chambers. 1977. *The nurse as group leader.* New York: Springer.

Clark, E. Louise. 1977. A model of nurse staffing. *Journal of Nursing Administration* 7,2:22–27.

Davis, Howard. 1971. *Planning for creative change in mental health services: a distillation of principles on research utilization.* Department of Health, Education and Welfare Publication No. HSM 73-9145. Washington, D.C.: U.S. Govt. Printing Office.

Dr. Finley versus the hospitals. 1977. *New York Times,* March 6, p. 4.

Dunn, J. D.; and Stevens, Elvis C. 1972. *Management of personnel: manpower management and organizational behavior.* New York: McGraw-Hill.

Frey, Mary. 1976. Planning for nursing service. *Hospital Progress* (October): 78–81.

Ganong, Warren; and Ganong, Joan Mary. 1974. Motivation and innovations: concerns for nursing administration. In *Motivating personnel and managing conflict.* Wakefield, Mass.: Contemporary Publishing.

Henry, Porter. 1975. Manage your sales force as a system. *Harvard Business Review* 53,2:85–94.

Housley, Charles E. 1976. Budgeting at the supervisor's level. *Hospital Topics* (March–April): 6–11.

Johnson, Richard; Kast, Fremont E; and Rosenzweig, James E. 1973. *The theory and management of systems,* 3rd ed. New York: McGraw-Hill.

Kafka, Vincent W. 1973. Every employee a winner. *Nursing Digest* 1,7:49–55.

Kast, Fremont E; and Rosenzweig, James E. 1974. *Organization and management: a systems approach,* 2nd ed. New York: McGraw-Hill.

Leininger, Madeleine. 1974. Conflict and conflict resolutions: theories and processes relevant to the health professions. *The American Nurse* (December): 17–22.

Lewis, Joyce H. 1976. Conflict management. *Journal of Nursing Administration* 6,10:18–22.

McCloskey, Joanne C. 1975. What rewards will keep nurses on the job? *American Journal of Nursing* 75,4:600–602.

Mager, Robert F. 1962. *Preparing instructional objectives.* Belmont, Calif.: Fearon Publishers.

Matsunaga, Grace. 1975. Nursing administrator must be chief initiator of needed change. *The American Nurse* (April): 10.

Peters, Joseph P. 1974. *Concept/commitment/action: a manual for planning programs and resources by health care institutions in New York City.* A joint publication of the United Hospital Fund of New York and the Health and Hospital Planning Council of Southern New York, Inc.

Pollock, Ted. 1971. *Managing others creatively.* New York: Hawthorne Books.

Ramey, Irene G. 1973. Eleven steps to proper staffing. *Nursing Digest* 1,7:4–8.

Sherwin, Douglas S. 1976. Management of objectives. *Harvard Business Review* 54,3:149–160.

Stevens, Barbara J. 1975. *The nurse as executive.* Wakefield, Mass.: Contemporary Publishing.

———. 1975. Management tools needed. *The American Nurse* (April): 9.

State governments and the social security administration seek new methods to reduce hospital costs. 1977. *New York Times,* February 27, pp. 1 and 38.

Strauss, George; and Sayles, Leonard R. 1972. *Personnel: the human problems of management,* 3rd ed. Englewood Cliffs, N.J.: Prentice-Hall.

Tannenbaum, Robert: Weschler, Irvin; and, Massarik, Fred. 1974. Leadership: a frame of reference. In *Small group communication,* 2nd ed., ed. Robert Cathcart and Larry Samovar. Dubuque, Iowa: William C. Brown.

Veninga, Robert. 1974. The management of conflict. In *Motivating personnel and managing conflict.* Wakefield, Mass.: Contemporary Publishing.

Chapter 4

Operations Research: A Quantitative Approach to Decision Making

Gus W. Grammas, William F. Clark, and Carolyn Chambers Clark

OBJECTIVES

After studying this chapter, the learner will:

- Define operations research
- List operations-research techniques
- Describe how operations-research techniques can be used by nurse-managers

DEFINITION

Operations research is best defined as the art and science of decision making. More elaborately, it is the application of the scientific method to tactical (operational) and strategic (long-term) problems in order to give management a quantitative basis for making decisions. Other areas of management analysis, such as accounting, finance, and market research, also develop quantitative material for making decisions, but the distinguishing characteristic of operations research is its use of the scientific method and advanced mathematical techniques to solve real problems. In order to emphasize the scientific aspect, some practitioners prefer the term "management science" rather than "operations research" (usually abbreviated as OR).

According to Craft and Langsford (1968, pp. 395–396), the scientific method consists of the following steps:

1   Understanding and defining| the nature of the problem that is to be solved.

2   Specifying the goals and objectives to be attained.

3   Specifying the assumptions and constraints of the problem.

4   Stating the resources to be used.

5   Gathering and analyzing the data.

6   Constructing a mathematical model designed to explain the observed facts and solve the problem.

7   Ascertaining whether or not the model is capable of explaining past experience and forecasting future performance.

8   Repeating the previous steps until a satisfactory model is constructed.

9   Using the model to solve the actual problem or forecast future performance.

In essence, the OR model is used to evaluate possible courses of action in order to determine which one would best accomplish a particular objective (for example, minimize costs).

Creativeness, or the art of operations research, is central to the development of the OR model. For example, it may be necessary to simplify complex mathematics in order to permit practical computation, or it may be desirable to use intelligent compromise in redefining the problem to be solved. In general, constructing an appropriate OR model requires judgment and experience as well as technical expertise.

Constructing a model is a technique of abstraction and simplification that permits the study of specific characteristics or systems under varying conditions. Models can be descriptive or explanatory. In OR, the word "model" means a mathematical or structural description of an activity. Models allow the operations researcher to manipulate the system represented in a variety of ways until a solution is found. Operations research allows for decision making in complex and uncertain situations, such as those that arise in the modern hospital or health care agency. For example, a mathematical model of hospital administration, client discharge, or nurse staffing can be manipulated more easily and efficiently than the actual administration, discharge, or staffing.

OPERATIONS RESEARCH AND HEALTH CARE SYSTEMS

There are great difficulties in developing mathematical models of health care systems because of the complexity of health services interactions and the lack of general agreement on classifications and definitions. Major problems in the modeling effort include the lack of established relationships between resource use and health conditions, the lack of agreed-upon measures of health status, and the large number of variables that must be included in any realistic representation of health services. Health services are now provided by a variety of institutions, independent practitioners, and governmental and private agencies. The interactions among these agencies are tenuous, and the separate services are regarded as autonomous. This results in a "nonsystem" that is so complex it even includes agencies with dual authorities, the prime example being the separation of administrative and medical or nursing authority in a hospital. A further problem confronting health modelers is that suitable measures of performance in a health service system, and data consistent with a systems representation, are difficult to obtain (Berg 1973; Fanshel and Bush 1970; and Torrance et al. 1972). Finally, inherent in the whole modeling effort is the number of dimensions in the health area; only the major variables can be considered, and many other relevant variables must be disregarded if the effort is to be at all feasible.

As Stimson and Stimson (1972) point out, the modeling effort places many responsibilities upon both the operations researcher and the manager of a health care system. The responsibilities of the researcher include: (1) defining the problem and not necessarily accepting what is stated by the manager; (2) determining what goals are being pursued by the manager (and the organization) and deciding whether or not to assist in the pursuit of these goals; (3) engaging in a mutual learning process with the manager (and others within the organization) so that all participants will be educated by the study; (4) building a model of the system in which the variables and the relationships among them are specified, and in which the relationships of the variables to the goals (the objective function) are clearly stated; (5) specifying the criteria by which alternatives will be ranked in order of preference and stating the method by which measurements will be made; (6) detailing how the data were generated, what possible errors they contain, and how these errors might affect the outcome of the study; and (7) including implementation of the results within the study, rather than leaving implementation up to someone else.

The responsibilities of the manager include: (1) differentiating among the various approaches of operations research; (2) specifying clearly why he or she is buying operations research and what he or she wants to achieve; (3) determining whether a particular study conducted in a particular way will actually help to achieve these goals; (4) committing the necessary resources, including his or her own time and effort; (5) working closely with the operations researcher once a study has been initiated; and (6) making sure that those in the organization who will be affected by the study have an opportunity to participate in it.

The use of operations-research techniques in the design, measurement, and control of health care delivery systems occurs at two levels. Most of the early work in this area concentrated on microanalytic studies, usually within hospitals. Much work has been done, for example, on generating mathematical models for scheduling outpatient clinics; staffing inpatient units of hospitals; analyzing the utilization of inpatient facilities; developing operating policies for blood banks; planning menus; and determining appropriate inventory-control methods for linens, drugs, and other consumables. More recently, operations-research models have been applied to macroanalytic studies, such as the design and operations of hospitals; regional planning of facilities for the delivery of health care; manpower planning in the health field; and computer information systems for quality and financial control in health care delivery. There is also much concern at present with the implementation problems of operations-research studies in the health area.

Mathematical models of health services date back to the early 1950s in the U.S. and even earlier in Great Britain (see, for example, Bailey 1952). Recently, several studies have provided an overview of the application of operations research to health care. Stimson and Stimson (1972) present an excellent review and critique of the literature on hospital related studies. Palmer (1975) provides a critique of a set of models he feels are most useful in estimating future effects of alternative proposals for improving health, including econometric and statistical methodologies, as well as the standard operations-research techniques. Shuman et al. (1975) analyze the progress in health applications from both the manager's and the researcher's perspectives, and organize a critique of these applications according to technique rather than area. Grosse (1972) discusses the application of analytical approaches to budgetary and legislative decisions in health policy at the level of the federal government. Finally, Fries (1976) provides an extensive bibliography on the applications of operations-research techniques to health care systems.

THE NURSE-MANAGER AND THE OPERATIONS RESEARCHER

This chapter is not meant to equip the nurse-manager to apply operations-research techniques. Rather, it is meant to familiarize the nurse-manager with the various ways in which operations research can assist health care delivery, and to discuss ways to interface the problems of the nurse-manager with the skills of the operations researcher.

First of all, it is necessary to define a decision problem. One way of classifying problems is to distinguish between those things that can be changed by the nurse-manager's direct action (controllable variables) and those that are outside managerial influence (environmental variables). Luck et al. (1972, pp. 57–59) specify the conditions of a decision problem that lends itself to an operations-research approach:

1 There is a decision maker who wants to attain a goal or make a change.

2 There are alternative ways to attain the goal, and these differ with respect to efficacy, the inherent risks, the resources to be used, and so on.

3 There are criteria for choice based upon some priority system. (operations researchers deal with numbers and models, not with values and priorities. The latter are within the nurse-manager's domain).

Once these conditions have been met, the nurse-manager should distinguish between the presenting symptoms and the decision problem. It may be necessary to obtain comparative statistics or conduct attitude surveys to determine the need for change.

Formulating the problem is the first and most important stage in an operations-research project. It is not unusual for operation researchers to encounter considerable suspicion and resistance in hospitals (Luck et al. 1971, pp. 59–60). Some problems can be defined quite easily, for example, how to obtain space for an ICU, or how large a new building ought to be. More complex issues, such as whether an ICU or new building should be built, present stickier definition problems. The operations researcher may ask the nurse-manager the following questions:

1 Are you willing to accept the proposed change?

2 Are there alternative ways to achieve the desired ends?

3 Are there priorities for choosing an appropriate action?

4 Are there data from which to construct hypotheses or draw conclusions?

5 If no data are available, how detailed must the data we collect be?

6 How large a sample is needed?

7 How reliable are the data?

8 What measures would most clearly represent the problem or the choices to be made?

9 How can a scale be constructed so that there is a good relationship between the actions of decision-makers and the operations-research model?

10 How can data that have been collected over a period of years best be used to forecast trends?

Nurse-managers who hope to work effectively with operations researchers must realize that it takes time to formulate and solve problems properly. There may be a large number of decision-makers and more time may need to be allocated to discussing conclusions in order to achieve acceptance and implementation. Technical jargon can create barriers. The nurse-manager and operation researcher must find a common language. New operations-research techniques may need to be developed. Some potential areas for joint nurse-manager–operations researcher work are: clinical problems, creating models of total systems of health care, relationships between hospitals and other health care delivery agencies, pooling resources or merging health care delivery (sub)systems, problems of continuity of care, retention of employees, educating governing boards and physicians on management problems, expansion problems, possible effects of public utility-type regulations on the hospital, possible effects of HSAs and noninstitutional health care services on the hospital (and vice versa).

TECHNIQUES OF ANALYSIS AND AREAS OF APPLICATION

In order to furnish the nurse-manager with some insight into the tools of operations research, the following techniques and areas of application will be discussed: linear programming, statistics and probability theory, queuing theory, inventory theory, computers and management information systems, design and operations of hospitals, gaming, and network analysis.

Linear Programming

This is a technique for specifying how to use limited resources to attain a specific objective, such as least cost or least time, when the available resources have alternate uses. This technique is the simplest of the constrained optimization models; it requires that the objective and constraints be stated as linear functions of the controllable variables.

Linear programming can be used to assign different classification of nursing personnel to different tasks; and to determine the best inventory strategy for hospital supplies, the best location of a new care unit, the least expensive yet most nutritious meals, the most efficient client care materials, the most effective brand of disinfectant, and whether to repair old equipment or purchase new equipment. For examples of solutions, see: Baligh and Laughhunn (1969) or Warner and Prawha (1972). Without linear programming techniques, these decisions must be based on experience or intuition (Johnson et al. 1973, p. 206). One disadvantage of the technique is that it cannot deal effectively with nonlinear conditions over time, but operations researchers are developing two techniques to offset this disadvantage: nonlinear and dynamic programming. One advantage of linear programming is that it forces the nurse-manager to clarify the aims of the particular system or subsystem.

Statistics and Probability Theory

These are useful in analyzing data and providing descriptive statistics. Operations researchers have developed ways to use statistical techniques to assist the decision-making process; this is done primarily by estimating parameters and testing hypotheses. Many managerial decisions relate to future events, many of which are not controllable. It is important for nurse-managers to understand the nature of probability theory and its use in decision making (Grier 1976). When there is a sequence of future events and each has a probability distribution, the nurse-manager can only act on intuition unless there is a systematic approach to account for all pertinent aspects. It might be helpful for the nurse-manager to address the following probabilities: What are the chances that nurses will receive back injuries while working on an orthopedic unit? What is the probable need for delivery rooms in an obstetric unit? What are the chances that the nursing staff will have to be increased or decreased at certain times of the day, week, or year?

One disadvantage of statistics and probability theory is that there may be a sampling error which can lead to a spurious correlation or invalid conclusion (Johnson et al. 1973, pp. 209–210). Random sampling is used to estimate probabilities and parameters, but how random is random? The following questions pertain to this difficulty: If every nth nurse is observed, what sampling error will there be? If contamination is measured on every nth sterile package, what will the sampling error be? If every nth nurse and client require x hours to complete prenatal teaching, what about the sampling error? Working with an operations researcher, the nurse-manager can help to reduce the sampling error to a minimum.

Queuing Theory

Queuing, or waiting line, theory is useful in decision making with respect to irregular demands for service. Costs are incurred in the length of the waiting line and the time lost in waiting, and queuing theory provides a useful way to deal with these costs. Since arrivals at outpatient clinics, emergency rooms, walk-in clinics, or general surgery may be random, sometimes there is insufficient staff and space to meet the demand, and at other times the staff sit by idly (Haussmann 1970). Some of the factors that may vary from problem to problem are: size of the client population being served, how patient the clientele is, the distribution of waiting and servicing times, the time pattern of arrivals, and the number of service units or providers (Johnson et al. 1973, pp. 210–211).

Outpatient clinics have been widely studied by queuing theorists and computer simulationists. They found that clients are usually on time for their appointments whereas doctors are usually late. With the increased work of clinical nurse specialists and nurse practitioners, nurse-managers might use operations-research techniques to demonstrate how nurses could be used more efficiently than tardy doctors.

Since 1950, staffing has been studied extensively by operations researchers. Operations-research techniques have been used to develop direct care indexes, which are now used to estimate the number of hours of direct nursing care that is required in each unit each day to meet predetermined standards of care (Stimson and Stimson 1972, pp. 9–14).

Inventory Theory

This has provided the framework for operations-research studies in blood banking, menu planning, and supply stocking. The basic objective of an inventory system is to meet the demand for an item at minimum cost (Pegels and Jelmert 1970). Decisions that must be made are when to buy items, how much to buy, and from which source. A mathematical model can be constructed that links a measure of effectiveness with the variables under control and those not under the control of the decision-maker (Agee et al. 1976, pp. 198–227). Computerized inventory control and information systems have been developed for regional blood banking. Such regionalization permits blood to be transferred among hospitals, decreasing the amount that becomes outdated. Historical data on supply and demand enable the administrator to plan for future blood needs and more efficient donor callup (Stimson and Stimson 1972, pp. 21–23).

Another approach to controlling inventory is the use of regression analysis to relate linear usage to the number of patients requiring intensive care (Stimson and Stimson 1972, p. 24). By combining data on the nursing staff with linen needs, a nurse-manager can work with an operations researcher to reduce linen inventory. To apply inventory theory, the nurse-manager would have to be able to get information on the past usage rates of individual stock items by the day, week, or month. Carrying costs, ordering costs, and the costs of shortages would have to be determined; these computations would probably require the most thought. There are advantages and disadvantages to inventory studies. Inventories can usually be reduced without affecting performance; although a study will provide data not previously available, such a study can be costly and may not be worth the money saved.

Computers and Management Information Systems

Another important area of operations research is the use of computers to build total hospital or agency information systems. Many companies are offering varied computerized applications to hospitals. Political and consumer pressures have forced health care delivery systems to reduce hospital costs. There is some hope that computers can bring about greater efficiency and therefore lower costs (Norwood et al. 1976). These pressures may lead to further attempts to control costs through automation and to justify hospital activities by means of operations research and systems analysis. Although there is more interest in this area (Stimson and Stimson 1972, pp. 26–28), there are difficulties in installing and using computers (Humphrey 1970, pp. 88–98).

It is possible to purchase accounting packages for hospital business offices and to install automated medical records. However, unresolved problems in these areas include ensuring unique patient identification, guaranteeing the confidentiality of information, and working out the technical problems of file construction. Computers could be used to a greater extent for planning and forecasting, for example, in determining the appropriate size of a planned ICU or rape crisis center.

Since little research has been done on the cost benefits of computerization, it is difficult to justify their use on cost savings alone. However, labor costs would seem to justify their use (Barnett 1971, pp. 55–57). As costs drop, hospitals and operations researchers will probably make greater use of computers.

More clients and more procedures are creating information problems. The proliferation of paperwork and labor hours is focusing attention on management information systems. Some operations researchers are suggesting that remote video terminals be located throughout large health care delivery systems to allow immediate access to client records. Less ambitious communication systems are linking the admitting office, nurses' station, laboratory, x-ray department, pharmacy, business office, and so forth by means of prepunched cards that transmit routine messages efficiently (Stimson and Stimson 1972, pp. 30–31). Luck et al. (1971, pp. 157–171) describe the design and structure of an information system pertaining to the admission and discharge of clients; basically it deals with the coordination and control of waiting lists, admissions, discharges, and management review. The purpose is to obtain data on these day-to-day decisions so that they can be reviewed periodically by managers. One purpose of data collection is to predict future workload so that appropriate steps can be taken to handle it within acceptable limits. It is believed that computer-operations-research techniques can effectively solve the problems of nursing staff allocation, nursing workload, nursing student training programs, nurse recruitment, and quality of care.

Design and Operations of Hospitals

Operations researchers have attempted to build models of hospitals. For example, Felter and Thompson (1969, pp. 450–462) tried to understand how special care units affect total system (hospital) operation. The paths followed by clients through a hospital, the probabilities for each path, and the means and standard deviations of the time spent in the various care zones were used to develop a simulation. The probability of bed use in each care unit was used to develop a model to maximize bed utilization. The computer allows decision-makers to work with more variables and more complex variables than could be remembered or written down on paper. The computer can store and retrieve information so quickly that both the whole system, the subsystems, and the interactions among parts and wholes can be studied (see, for example, Barnoon and Wolfe [1968]).

Computer simulation is used for the following: to predict the consequences of changes in policies, conditions, or methods without spending money for or risking actual change; to learn more about the system so it can be redesigned or refined; to allow the staff to become familiar with forthcoming or expected situations that are not yet available in the real-life environment; and to demonstrate the chances of success (Johnson et al. 1973, pp. 214–215). Several noncomputer simulations have been developed for use by nurse-managers; for example, *You are Barbara Jordan* (1970) is a simulation exercise to help nurse-managers appraise and act on twenty-four items of written communication, ranging from routine staff scheduling problems to emergency situations.

Gaming

Some of the significant problems the nurse-manager may have to deal with include contending with a complex environment *and* making decisions in competition with other managers. Simulation of these competitive situations is called *gaming*. So far, these simulations have been used primarily for training and not for research or analysis. Some research has been done on the human relations aspects of decision making (Johnson et al. 1973, pp. 213–214). The interaction among members of a nursing team or health care team is a fruitful area for research. Luck et al. (1971, pp. 114–130) report the use of a game as both a training and a research device; it is meant to train doctors and nurses to manage a unit and to study the decision-making processes in managing a 120-bed general hospital unit. The game has two players or teams of players, one representing the doctor and the other the nurse-manager. There are game administrators who work out the effects of the players' decisions and provide emergency admissions and additions to the waiting list. The participants must make specific decisions. While the participants play the game, operations researchers collect statistics and attempt to discover the implicit and explicit rules used by the participants to make decisions.

Network Analysis

This is a managerial technique that is used to predict or identify the performance of a subsystem; its purpose is to design, coordinate, or control.

Each subsystem or link is described in relation to other parts or activities of the system, and a visual representation outlines the task.

There are both simple and complex forms of network analysis. Some have general applications, while others are for specific types of projects. Critical-path scheduling (to complete a project in minimum time or with minimum cost) is a basic concept in network analysis.

PERT (program evaluation review technique) is a widely used type of network analysis. The advantages of PERT techniques in the management of complex research and development activities are to identify the sequence and relationships of significant events, to measure and identify the relative uncertainty in meeting various activities, to identify and plan for critical and noncritical time factors, and to be able to compute the current probability for meeting scheduled dates. In some network analyses, tradeoff decisions in terms of cost versus time can also be identified. In complex systems computers are almost invariably required (Johnson et al. 1973, pp. 244–266). Network analysis could be applied in the following areas: planning and developing auditing systems, integrating and coordinating budgets, determining priorities in the acquisition and timing of capital purchases, installing and making the conversion to computer systems, scheduling unusual operations or procedures, long-range planning, revising or installing a management reporting system, and starting up emergency or standby facilities.

PROBLEMS IN IMPLEMENTATION

The techniques of operations research offer a great deal in the analysis of health care systems. It must be acknowledged, however, that there are many shortcomings in the operations-research studies discussed here so that they have not been fully implemented. From the manager's viewpoint, this lack of implementation may be due to any of the following (Stimson and Stimson, 1972): (1) omission of certain problems deemed important by administrators, (2) the tendency to view the hospital as a separable system, (3) the tendency to view the health system as mechanistic, (4) omission of the medical staff from hospital studies, (5) omission of the client from hospital studies, (6) failure to foresee dysfunctional consequences of introducing computer-based technology, (7) failure to assess the complexities of applying computer-based technology, (8) insufficient attention to model building and to the way in which data for models are generated, (9) omission of variables that are difficult to quantify, (10) failure to include detailed information on the costs and benefits of proposed changes, (11) failure to recognize limitations on the power of the manager, and (12) failure to read the literature on implementation. Certainly, improved methods, techniques, and tools are needed for the analysis of health care systems.

SUMMARY

Operations research holds great potential for management. Although there are difficulties in creating mathematical models of health care systems, nurse-managers need to be able to identify areas where they can work with operations researchers on solutions to health care problems. Some of the techniques that can be applied are linear programming, statistics and probability theory, queuing theory, inventory theory, computers and management information systems, design and operations of hospitals, gaming, and network analysis. This chapter is meant to give the nurse-manager a broad overview of the skills an operations researcher can offer, using a systems approach to help identify appropriate decision-making questions.

REFERENCES

Agee, Marvin H.; Taylor, Robert E.; and Torgersen, Paul E. 1976. *Quantitative analysis for management decisions*. Englewood Cliffs, N.J.: Prentice-Hall.

Barker, J. 1971. Computers in hospitals. *The Hospital* 67 (August): 279–282.

Bailey, N. T. J. 1952. Operational research in medicine. *Operational Research Quarterly* 3:24–29.

Baligh, H. H.; and Laughhunn, D. L. 1969. An economic and linear model of the hospital. *Health Services Research* 4,4:293–303.

Ball, Marion J. 1971. An overview of total medical information systems. *Methods of Information in Medicine* 10 (April): 73–82.

Barnett, G. 1971. Can computers reduce manpower needs? *Hospitals, J.A.H.A.* 45 (August 16): 55–57.

Barnoon, S.; and Wolfe, H. 1968. Scheduling a multiple operating room system: a simulation approach. *Health Services Research* 3,4:272–285.

Berg, R. L., ed. 1973. *Health status indexes*. Chicago: Hospital Research and Educational Trust.

Catassi, C. A.; and Peterson, E. L. 1967. The blood inventory control system—helping blood bank management through computerized inventory control. *Transfusion* 7 (January–February): 60–69.

Craft, C. J.; and Langsford, G. L. 1968. Operations research. In *Systems and procedures: a handbook for business and industry,* 2nd ed., ed. V. Lazzaro. Englewood Cliffs, N.J.: Prentice-Hall, pp.423.

Duckett, Stephen. 1977. Nurse rostering with game theory. *Journal of Nursing Adminstration* (January):58–59.

Fanshel, S.; and Bush, J. W. 1970. A health-status index and its application to health-services outcomes. *Operations Research* 18,6:1021–1066.

Fries, B. E. 1976. Bibliography of operations research in health care systems. *Operations Research* 24,5:801–814.

Grier, M. R. 1976. Decisionmaking about patient care. *Nursing Research* 25,2:105–110.

Grosse, R. N. 1972. Analysis in health planning. In *Analysis of public systems,* ed. A. W. Drake, R. L. Keeney, and P. M. Morse. Cambridge, Mass.: M.I.T. Press, pp. 401–428.

Haussmann, R. K. D. 1970. Waiting time as an index of quality of nursing care. *Health Services Research* 5,2:92–105.

Humphrey, M. O. 1970. A reappraisal of computer utilization. *Hospital Progress* 51:88–98.

Johnson, Richard A.; Kast, Fremont; and Rosenzweig, James E. 1973. Quantitative techniques of analysis. In *The theory and management of systems.* New York: McGraw-Hill, pp. 193–273.

Luck, G. M.; Luckman, J.; Smith, B. W.; and Stringer, J. 1971. *Patients, hospitals, and operational research.* London: Tavistock Institute of Human Relations.

Mariner, E. T. 1971. Hospitals haven't realized potential of data processing. *Hospital Financial Management* 25 (February):3–5.

Norwood, D. D.; Hawkins, R. E.; and Gall, J. E., Jr. 1976. Information system benefits hospital, improves patient care. *Hospitals, J.A.H.A.* 50,18:79–83.

Palmer, B. A. 1975. Models in planning and operating health services. In *A guide to models in governmental planning and operations,* ed. S. I. Gass and R. L. Sisson. Potomac, Md.: Sauger Books, pp. 347–374.

Pegels, C. C.; and Jelmert, A. E. 1970. An evaluation of blood-inventory policies: a Markov chain application. *Operations Research* 18,6:1087–1098.

Poland, Marilyn. 1970. A system for assessing and meeting patient care needs. *American Journal of Nursing* 70,7:1479–1482.

Shuman, L. J.; Speas, R. D., Jr.; and Young, J. P., eds. 1975. *Operations research in health care.* Baltimore, Md.: Johns Hopkins University Press.

Somers, June B. 1971. A computerized nursing care system. *Hospitals, J.A.H.A.* 45 (April 16): 93–100.

Stimson, David H.; and Stimson, Ruth H. 1972. *Operations research in hospitals: diagnosis and prognosis.* Chicago: Hospital Research and Educational Trust.

Torrance, G. W.; Thomas, W. H.; and Sackett, D. L. 1972. A utility maximization model for evaluation of health care programs. *Health Services Research* 7,2: 118–133.

Warner, D. M.; and Prawda, J. 1972. A mathematical programming model for scheduling nursing personnel in a hospital. *Management Science* 19,4:411–422.

You are Barbara Jordan. 1970. Chicago: Hospital Research and Educational Trust.

Chapter 5

Evaluation from the Home Health Agency Perspective

Rita DeCotiis and Joan Schroeder

OBJECTIVES

After studying this chapter, the learner will:

- Define evaluation
- Discuss one systematic process of evaluation
- Identify methodologies in evaluation

As the health care industry has grown and the costs have spiraled, it has become essential to have systematic methods for evaluating the delivery of health care. The system must have feedback mechanisms for regulating actions and evaluating outcomes. Today, as never before, the health system is accountable for its actions, and as accountability increases, the system must meet growing demands for care and provide the highest quality of clinical competence in a cost-effective manner.

DEFINITION AND OBJECTIVES OF EVALUATION

Evaluation is the identification and measurement of organization performance and results. Any structure, process, or outcome that is being evaluated should be judged against predetermined criteria or standards.

An evaluation of *structure* is a review of a setting or an organization. Examples of this type of evaluation include the National League for Nursing's accreditation program for home health agencies and the Joint Hospital Commission's program for evaluating hospitals. An evaluation of *process* is a review of professional performance by means of observation, record review, peer review, and client feedback. An evaluation of *outcome* is a review of the effectiveness of services rendered by means of statistical data, documentation of care, and client status and satisfaction.

The purpose of evaluation is to assess the appropriateness, adequacy, effectiveness, and efficiency of services. Appropriateness pertains to whether the services were utilized properly and whether the level of care

Table 5-1   Evaluation

Appropriateness

Is the home the best place fo the client to receive care?

Are the services provided at a proper level?

Example: Should a physical therapist be visiting regularly, or could restorative nursing be used under a physical therapy plan of care?

Adequacy

Are the necessary professional and paraprofessional services available so that a client can remain at home?

Are supportive community services available and included in the plan of care?

Example: A nurse visits twice weekly. The client was not receiving enough assistance and supervision on a daily basis.

A home health aide is needed 4 hours daily to assist with personal care, meals, rest, and an exercise regimen.

As recovery progresses and the client can better take care of himself or herself, the aide can be dismissed.

Meal delivery needs to be arranged so that the client can comply with the therapeutic diet.

Effectiveness

Are the goals specifically defined and measurable?

Is there evidence of client learning and compliance with such prescribed regimes as diet, medications, and exercise?

Example: A diabetic who understands the disease and its control will indicate this in his or her behavior and feedback of nursing instructions.

Efficiency

Are personnel and material utilized in the best way to control quality and costs?

Example: Time studies look at how much time a nurse spends for a home visit, as well as the activities that precede and follow the visit and travel.

Districting may decrease travel time and mileage costs.

Recordings made during a visit may decrease office time.

was suitable; adequacy refers to the resources the organization can provide to meet the needs of the community and individual client; effectiveness is the measure of how well these resources were put to use; and efficiency pertains to the productivity and costs. Table 5-1 presents evaluation questions.

SYSTEMATIC PROGRAM EVALUATION

One of the problems facing home health agencies today is the federal government's demand for a systematic and ongoing program of evaluation. Before the advent of Medicare, most agencies made evaluations only on an informal, undocumented, and infrequent basis. The gathering of statistical data, revision of policies and procedures, performance evaluation, and record review (to name only a few functions) were done only sporadically and in a way that did not show the relationships among them.

All aspects of a home health care program must be interrelated to provide the optimum service to the community. It is not an easy task to perfect a system of evaluation for this type of agency because of the many variables that exist when establishing measurable criteria.

The first step in planning for a systematic approach is to decide what group has responsibility for the overall assessment of the components. In many agencies, this task has been assigned to the professional advisory committee. This committee annually assesses the reports submitted to it by review teams and determines whether the stated objectives for the year have been met. At that time, the program objectives for the forthcoming year are established. These objectives should reflect the agency's plan to improve the quality of its services, implement new services to fill identified needs, and ensure efficient utilization of existing services.

There are many elements in program evaluation, and they vary according to the agency's size and program scope. Table 5-2 outlines the methodology used in one home health organization, Nursing Service, Incorporated, of Ridgewood, New Jersey. (This agency provides home health care and public health nursing to approximately 70,000 persons who reside in a five-town area. The professional staff consists of fifteen registered nurses, five physical therapists, two occupational therapists, and one speech therapist.)

Utilization Review in a Home Health Agency

Utilization review, or case record review (these terms are used interchangeably), is required of certified home health agencies in order to comply with Medicare's Conditions of Participation. This is another way of making the agency accountable for its actions to both the client who

Table 5-2   Utilization Review, Organization and Operations

Nursing Service, Incorporated
74 Passaic Street
Ridgewood, New Jersey 07451

I Organizational structure

   A BYLAWS
     1 Purpose   To ensure legal compliance through review
     2 Responsibility of   Bylaws Committee
     3 When done   Annually (October)

   B ARTICLES OF INCORPORATION
     1 Purpose   To show internal lines of responsibility
     2 Responsibility of   Professional Advisory Committee, Executive Director
     3 When done   Annually (June)

   C NONPROFIT STATUS
     1 Purpose   To show internal lines of responsibility
     2 Responsibility of   Professional Advisory Committee, Executive Director
     3 When done   Annually

   D ORGANIZATIONAL CHART
     1 Purpose   To show internal lines of responsibility
     2 Responsibility of   Professional Advisory Committee, Executive Director
     3 When done   Annually

   E AGENCY OBJECTIVE
     1 Purpose   To show internal lines of responsibility
     2 Responsibility of   Professional Advisory Committee, Executive Director
     3 When done   Annually

II Financial data

   A BUDGETS
     1 *Agency*
       a Purpose   To review and revise present year's budget and plan for next year.
       b Responsibility of   Finance Committee, Executive Director
       c When done   Annually (March)
     2 *United Fund*
       a Purpose   To review and revise present year's budget and plan for next year.

Table 5-2   Utilization Review, Organization and Operations (continued)

b Responsibility of	Finance Committee, Executive Director
c When done	Annually (July)
3 *United Way*	
a Purpose	To review and revise present year's budget and plan for next year
b Responsibility of	Finance Committee, Executive Director
c When done	Annually (October)
B <u>AUDIT</u>	
1 *Agency*	
a Purpose	Financial data examined by C.P.A. Authorized by the Board of Directors
b Responsibility of	Finance Committee
c When done	Annually (February)
2 *Medicare*	
a Purpose	To determine compliance with Medicare reimbursement regulations
b Responsibility of	Executive Director, Office Manager, Finance Committee
c When done	At fiscal intermediaries' discretion, annually
3 *Cost analysis*	
a Purpose	To determine and document costs
b Responsibility of	Finance Committee—C.P.A. Authorized by the Board of Directors
c When done	Annually (February)
4 *Fee scale*	
a Purpose	To adjust fees according to documented costs
b Responsibility of	Board of Directors, Executive Director
c When done	Annually (March)
C <u>STATISTICAL DATA</u>	
1 *Review of management information systems report*	
a Purpose	To determine quantity of service, population served, sources of referral, payment sources

Table 5-2   Utilization Review, Organization and Operations (continued)

b Responsibility of	Monthly: Executive Director. Annually: Executive Director and Planning Committee
c When done	Monthly: Annually (February)
2 *Review of discharge statistics*	
a Purpose	To determine statistics on discharge status
b Responsibility of	Executive Director
c When done	Annually (February)
D <u>TIME STUDY ANALYSIS</u>	
a Purpose	To determine average time per visit, to be used with the cost analysis study
b Responsibility of	Executive Director, C.P.A. Authorized by the Board of Directors
c When done	Annually (February)
E <u>POLICIES</u>	
1 *Medical policies*	
a Purpose	To provide safe medical direction for those responsible for client care
b Responsibility of	Professional Advisory Committee, Executive Director, Nursing and Therapy Staff
c When done	Annually (June)
2 *School health policies*	
a Purpose	To provide safe medical direction for those responsible for client care
b Responsibility of	Professional Advisory Committee, Executive Director, Nursing and Therapy Staff
c When done	Annually (June)

Table 5-2   Utilization Review, Organization and Operations (continued)

3 *School health policies*
   a Purpose — To provide safe school health policies for those responsible for school health programs

   b Responsibility of — Professional Advisory Committee, Executive Director, Nursing Personnel assigned to the schools

   c When done — Annually (June)

F PERSONNEL

1 *Review of personnel policies*
   a Purpose — To provide well-defined policies for agency and staff responsibilities

   b Responsibility of — Personnel Committee, Executive Director

   c When done — Annually (September)

2 *Job descriptions*
   a Purpose — To provide clear guidelines for areas of staff performances

   b Responsibility of — Personnel Committee, Executive Director

   c When done — Annually (September)

3 *Coordinated inservice programs*
   a Purpose — To provide an overall plan for a coordinated inservice program for the year that will meet the needs of the professional staff

   b Responsibility of — Executive Director, Professional Advisory Committee, Professional Staff

   c When done — Annually (September)

4 *Performance evaluation: new employees*
   a Purpose — To determine level of performance of employee

   b Responsibility of — Nursing Supervisor, Therapy Supervisor

Table 5-2 Utilization Review, Organization and Operations (continued)

c When done	Upon completion of 3 month's employment, then after 1 year's employment
5 *Staff*	
a Purpose	To determine level of performance of employee
b Responsibility of	Nursing Supervisor, Therapy Supervisor
c When done	Annually
G EVALUATION OF SERVICES	
1 *Disease program:* client care audit	
a Purpose	To determine areas that need improved quality of care
b Responsibility of	Committee from Nursing, Therapy Staff
c When done	Every month on 10 percent of the number of discharged patients. Annual summary (April)
2 *Utilization review*	
a Purpose	To determine if services are being utilized properly
b Responsibility of	Professional Advisory Committee, Nurse Reviewer
c When done	Quarterly (April, June, September, December)
3 *Client questionnaire*	
a Purpose	To elicit feedback from the consumer as to effectiveness, quality, and appropriateness of services rendered
b Responsibility of	Executive Director
c When done	Ongoing. Summaries reviewed annually
4 *Senior health consultation services*	
a Purpose	To determine adequacy and effectiveness of services in meeting objectives
b Responsibility of	Professional Advisory Committee, Executive Director, Professional Staff
c When done	Annually (December)
5 *School health program*	
a Purpose	To formulate plans to meet changing needs in the schools

Table 5-2   Utilization Review, Organization and Operations (continued)

b Responsibility of	Professional Advisory Committee, Executive Director, Professional Staff
c When done	Annually (December)
6 *Disease prevention and health supervision*	
a Purpose	To determine effectiveness of program and anticipate future needs of the community
b Responsibility of	Professional Advisory Committee, Professional Staff
c When done	Annually (September)—3 months before renewal of municipal contracts
7 *Child health conference*	
a Purpose	To determine utilization and effectiveness of the program
b Responsibility of	Professional Advisory Committee, Professional Staff
c When done	Annually (December)
H REVIEW OF RECOMMENDATIONS	
a Purpose	To improve services by implementing recommendations of the State Department of Health
b Responsibility of	Professional Advisory Committee
c When done	Annually
1 *State department of health recertification survey*	
a Purpose	To improve services by implementing recommendations of the State Department of Health
b Responsibility of	Board of Directors
c When done	Annually (January)
2 *Fiscal intermediary compliance review*	
a Purpose	To determine areas for improvement so that agency can conform to requirements of Medicare and Medicaid
b Responsibility of	Professional Advisory Committee (December). Board of Directors (January)
c When done	Annually

receives care and the government, which funds a large share of the cost. The Federal Register states that this evaluation must be made at least quarterly on a percentage of both active and closed clinical records to make sure that services are being rendered according to established policies. An ongoing review must be made on the clinical records of clients who have been with the agency more than 60 days so that appropriateness and continuation of care can be assessed. Utilization review can reveal gaps in services. The review committee of one agency that examined the record of a client found that a qualified social worker needed to be added to the health team. The multitude of social and economic problems as shown in the family profile and client problem list was a deterrent to rehabilitation. The committee's recommendations were brought to the agency board, and negotiations were begun to secure a social worker on a contractual basis. It should be stressed that all recommendations resulting from the utilization review must be acted upon, and a report of the agency administration's action must be submitted to the committee. Overutilization of professional services may point out the reluctance of a nurse or therapist to discontinue service. For example, a client with cardiac disease should be monitored by the nurse only until this condition stabilizes. Yet an important aspect of case management is assisting the client or the family to find solutions to other problems that have been identified in the nursing assessment. This should be done during the period when the nurse is making visits since future planning should not require a continuation of nursing visits. Table 5-3 shows a utilization review summary and report.

The review committee in a nonprofit voluntary agency is appointed by the board of directors after consultation with the executive director and members of the staff. It is a multidisciplinary committee, composed of those who provide services as well as consumers. This group should include at least a public health nurse, a physician, a representative of each of the therapeutic services provided by the agency, a staff member, and a consumer. After the committee is selected, each member must receive an in-depth introduction to the policies, procedures, and philosophy of the agency. Each committee member must also understand the utilization review process and its role in promoting change in the home health care system.

In the agencies where the authors work the review is performed by the entire advisory committee. The agency administration has suggested that a subcommittee be formed, but the advisory group rejected this proposal because they feel that they are better informed since they have taken part in the review process. The records are read, measured against a set of criteria, and evaluated by a objective reviewer. The objectivity of the

Table 5-3 Utilization Review, Summary and Report

Nursing Service, Incorporated
74 Passaic Street
Ridgewood, New Jersey 07451
September 13, 1976

Method of Selection

Random sample of all new admissions, July–August 1976

Number Reviewed

19 cases were reviewed—3 cases having multidisciplinary visits, bringing total review to 22.

Total admissions: 92

Size of sample: 22

Percentage of all admissions July and August reviewed: 24

Utilization Problems Identified and Recommendations

1 When the physician's written plan of treatment is delayed in reaching the agency contact the physician and reinforce the need for written orders.

2 Review the need for documented communications between nurses and therapists at staff conferences.

3 Case no. 0002204 —Need for services of a medical social worker because of ongoing marital and financial problems.

4 Case no. 000154 — Overutilization of services. Skilled nursing no longer needed. Client should be assisted to find a lower level of care and community resources. Example: Community meals and a bath service. Nursing to be discontinued.

Action Taken on Recommendations

1 Notice is to be attached to all physician's plans of treatment and requests for recertification of orders stating that the form must be completed and returned to the agency within 5 days.

2 Documentation of conferences on multidisciplinary cases was discussed at a staff meeting.

3 Negotiations are now under way toward signing a contract with Family Counseling to utilize a qualified social worker for home visits.

4 Client was referred to Community Meals and Visiting Homemakers to meet the present needs. Discharged from this agency.

---

reviewer is an extremely important consideration for effective evaluation. Many agencies have found that a professional from another home health agency can be more objective in analyzing the records than an employee of their own organization. Every case record that is over the 60-day period is automatically reviewed by an agency supervisor before sending a request for recertification of orders to a physician. Table 5-4 illustrates the policies used for case record review in one home health agency.

Table 5-4   Case Record Review Process in One Home Health Agency

Purpose

To improve the quality, availability, and appropriateness of health services rendered to clients and families in the community.

Objectives

The objectives of the Case Record Review Process are:

- to measure the availability of services against the needs of the clients
- to determine the appropriate use of service in duration and level of care
- to identify gaps in service
- to identify areas for staff development and coordination
- to determine degree of continuity of care

Designation of Responsibility

The Board of Directors of Nursing Service, Inc., has designated the Professional Advisory Committee as the responsible body to perform utilization review either through the full committee or an appointed subcommittee. The subcommittee will consist of a physician, a consumer, and a representative of each of the professional services provided by the agency.

Functions of the Committee

1 A public health nurse reviewer who is not an employee of the agency will be selected and given responsibility for the initial review of client records. This nurse will then complete a review form and present the preliminary review findings to the committee.

2 The committee will review each case presented and make recommendations to the Executive Director.

3 At its next meeting, the committee will review all actions taken on its prior recommendations.

Selection of Cases

1 A random sample of at least 10 percent of all active and discharged case records will be reviewed each year.

2 Records of all clients who have been receiving services for 60 days will be reviewed prior to recertification of orders from the physician. This review will be an ongoing one, performed by a nurse or therapist functioning in a supervisory capacity.

3 Problem cases may be referred for utilization review by any staff member.

4 All cases determined ineligible for reimbursement by third party payees will be reviewed.

Committee Report and Recommendations

A report of the committee's findings and recommendations will be submitted to the Executive Director for action, and staff personnel will be apprised of the report. Actions taken on the recommendations will be submitted to the committee prior to the next meeting.

STAFF PERFORMANCE EVALUATION

Job satisfaction is an important element in encouraging clinical competency and productivity, and so the review of staff performance is an integral part of evaluating the quality of care being given in a health care system. It is also a method of assessing the employees' potentialities to make sure that they are being maximized. Every health care facility should establish policies for personnel evaluation, including the standards for measurement and a decision as to who will apply these standards. This is a mutual process in which the staff members should also have the opportunity to measure their own performance in terms of agency policies.

Table 5-5 is an evaluation form used by the Visiting Nurses of Northern Bergen County, Incorporated, Mahwah, New Jersey.

Client satisfaction with the services received should also enter into the performance evaluation. Keeping an anecdotal record in each employee's file of feedback from consumers provides valuable information when assessing performance. The supervisor who receives a routine call from a client and, in the course of conversation, is told of the exemplary performance of a staff member should note this. Notes on specific job behavior should also be put into the file. These notes should be objective, pointing out strengths and weaknesses. When an employee is found lacking in an area, documentation of methods used to improve the performance and the outcome must be noted. For instance, the nurse who has difficulty in counseling the terminally ill client's family may need further guidance on the subject of death and dying. The supervisor should assess how much professional growth has taken place after such assistance has been given.

The results of peer review discussed later in this chapter must also be taken into account when evaluating staff performance. The employee who does not interact constructively with other professionals in the system can be viewed as a liability to the agency. Performance evaluation is extremely important in reaching the goal of providing quality home health care. It is a tool by which the administrator can judge not only the areas of competence but those that need development on either a group or individual basis.

PROFESSIONAL AUDITS

Evaluation of nursing care includes auditing nursing actions by observation or record review. Standards of practice must be developed and used as the criteria for measurement. Maria Phaneuf's *The Nursing Audit— Profile for Excellence* (1972) has been applied, with minor revisions, to many community health nursing agencies. It is based on seven functions

Table 5-5 Evaluation Form

EMPLOYEE _____	Date of appointment to present position _____
POSITION TITLE _____	Date of evaluation _____

Directions for completing form:
This form is for appraising and discussing an employee's performance in his or her present position. Completed form will supply information for advising the employee on his or her performance and for planning development activities with and for the employee. Description should be completed first; then check the appropriate block to indicate degree of performance. The completed form should be retained in the employee's personnel file.

RATE BY LETTER:	U — Unsatisfactory	F — Fair	G —Good
	VG — Very Good	E — Excellent	

	Job performance and factors affecting job performance		Rating	Remarks
1	PRODUCTIVITY	Ability to get the job done, degree to which employee accomplishes specified job duties, responsibilities, and objectives.		
	Quantity	Industry or application.		
	Quality	Accuracy, completeness, and efficiency.		
2	RELATIONSHIPS WITH OTHERS	Effectiveness in working with clients, coworkers, and public.		
3	KNOWLEDGE OF WORK	Understanding of all phases of his or her work and related matters.		
4	PLANNING AND ORGANIZING	Ability to plan ahead, schedule, and lay out work. Safe and effective use of personnel, materials, and equipment.		
5	JUDGMENT	Ability to size up a problem, get and evaluate the facts, reach sound conclusions, and present them effectively.		
		Willingness to make decisions, and the degree to which decisions or actions are sound.		

Table 5-5   Evaluation Form (continued)

			Rating	Remarks
6	ADAPTABILITY	Quickness to grasp, interpret, and adjust to instructions, new situations, methods, and procedures.		
7	INITIATIVE	Ability to originate or develop ideas and to get things started.		
8	SELF-EXPRESSION	Ability to communicate thoughts orally and in writing.		
9	LEADERSHIP AND DEVELOPMENT OF PERSONNEL	Ability to set objectives, maintain communication, and instill in others the desire to accomplish objectives. Recognition and development of the aptitudes, abilities, and capacities of others.		
10	DESCRIBE ANY OTHER FACTORS AFFECTING HIS OR HER PERFORMANCE (e.g., tact, poise, common sense, discretion, dependability, attitude, appearance, punctuality, attendance, personal and professional integrity).			

Overall performance

11   Indicate overall performance by check: _____ Unsatisfactory
_____ Fair   _____ Good (standard meets requirements)
_____ Very Good   _____ Excellent

On what specific items (1–10 do you feel improvements could be made?

What actions do you plan to suggest to help bring about these improvements (employer or employee action)?

Describe any change in performance or progress since last appraisal.

Prepared by _____ in consultation with _____ who knows of person appraised.

Development, discussion, summary

12   Concerning employee's development in present assignment: What did you learn about this employee's desires, ambitions, job preferences, attitudes, self-development activities?

What development activities were planned with and for the employee to help him or her develop on these factors?

On what factors was it agreed to try and improve?

Table 5-5   Evaluation Form (continued)

Reviewed with employee on: Date _____

Signature _____

Title _____

**EMPLOYEE'S STATEMENT OF REACTION TO
EVALUATION**

Date _____Signature _____

of professional nursing that were identified by Lesnik and Anderson (Phaneuf 1972, p. 5):

1 Application and execution of the physician's legal orders.
2 Observation of symptoms and reactions.
3 Supervision of the client.
4 Supervision of those, other than physicians, who are participating in care.
5 Reporting and recording.
6 Application and execution of nursing procedures and techniques.
7 Promotion of physical and emotional health by direction and teaching.

There are fifty components and scores that range from excellent to unsafe. Phaneuf notes that six are exercised independently, while only the first is dependent upon the physician. Third-party payers (especially Medicare, with its definition of skilled nursing care) seem to judge eligibility on a technical task basis, while this audit appraises nursing judgment, ability in case management, scientific knowledge and its application, and teaching skills. This audit is limited, however, by its disease orientation, which does not make it as useful for family health supervision—an integral aspect of community health nursing. A record is a very helpful evaluation tool in this field because proper documentation assures continuity and ongoing reassessments.

Physical therapy is beginning to develop criteria and audit methodology pertinent to home care, as shown in the work of Samuel Feitelberg (1975) at the University of Vermont Medical Center. A task force of the Home Health Agency Assembly of New Jersey and the New Jersey Occupational Therapy Association has developed guidelines and criteria for the utilization of occupational therapy (1976). These guidelines are an important contribution to the team approach for the client and are a valuable resource for the development of an occupational therapy audit.

Auditing the outcome of client care requires specific diagnostic groups with similiar problems and needs. The Joint Commission on Accreditation of Hospital Auditing and Improving Patient Care focuses on outcomes. The Quality Assurance Project of the Pennsylvania Assembly of Home Health Agencies (under a Health, Education and Welfare Regional Medical Program grant) designed a client care audit system for quality assessment. This has some excellent features, including examples of criteria specific to home health agencies. The ten diagnostic categories most prevalent in agency caseloads were identified through a representative sample of agencies; these include: diabetes mellitus on insulin, cerebrovascular accident, chronic obstructive lung disease, congestive heart disease, hip fracture, postcataract surgery, arthritis, cardiovascular disease, cancer of colon with colostomy, and mental illness. Health supervision has been included, with categories of comprehensive care for an adult client and maternal and child health—antepartum, postpartum, and infant. Exceptions to each criterion are suggested, as are suggestions for the management of critical complications. Their method of audit also includes examination of discharged records. A valuable component is the inclusion of the multidisciplinary professional team. For example, the CVA category includes nursing, physical, occupational, and speech therapies. This is particularly helpful because there is a paucity of available material on goal-setting and continuing care in speech therapy. In the report, Berkoben (1976, p. 5) states that process criteria could be developed for concurrent auditing. Agencies could use either retrospective auditing (examination of patient care records after discharge), concurrent auditing (examination of records while care is outgoing), or a combination of these.

The American Nurses Association's Standards for Nursing Services include integration of the nursing care programs into the total program of the health care organization. Rotkovich (1976, p. 34) urges a quality assurance program for each discipline to use in evaluating its own performance. These programs could then be reviewed by one quality assurance committee in evaluating total patient care. Although this approach, with its holistic perspective, seems logical, it may be difficult to establish in the physician-oriented institution. Professional boundaries continue to be rigid, which results in fragmentation of services to the client. Some home health agencies are attempting to implement a multidisciplinary approach to health care. In such agencies, the physician is not dominant, and the plan of treatment could be more team-centered. However, not having enough physician participation is a limitation. Thus, where there is more freedom and independent practice for nurses and other health professionals, there may be less coordination, communication, and cooperation with the physician in providing community health services. This is often brought to light in both audits and utilization reviews. Audits often point out incomplete diagnoses and medical histories obtained from the physician or referring hospital. In those cases, the professional who is providing care in the home does not have the necessary information to make a total assessment. This would be true in a case where a nurse is requested to treat a fecal impaction without being told that the patient had a serious cardiac condition. Closing the communication gaps in the health care system leads to a higher quality of service. Crossing the interface among health disciplines is essential in providing quality care to the consumer.

EVALUATION STUDIES AND ADMISSION REVIEWS

The kinds of evaluation studies and admissions reviews that are made in hospitals *are not yet required* for home health agencies, but they probably will be in the future. Such valuable assessments of potential problem areas may include statistical reports of patterns and deviations rather than subjectively perceived reports. Furthermore, such assessments focus on groups rather than on individuals. Kleffel offers a wide range of home health subjects that could be assessed, including: the quality of teaching and supervision; clients' compliance with therapeutic diets; the adequacy of weekend services; indicators of change in the level of care needed by clients; the frequency and reason for readmission; and the effectiveness of discharge planning. The procedure for developing a home health evaluation study includes: the selection of subjects, development of methodology and sampling, delegation of assignments with completion date (usually short term), collection of data, presentation of findings to a utilization review committee, followup of recommendations from the committee, and reevaluation (Kleffel 1972, pp. 69–75.) Although this type of study is not presently mandated for home health agencies, it is most compatible with utilization reviews and outcome audits, and its influence on the total system of evaluation would be significant. For example, a study of the adequacy of weekend services or need for 24-hour coverage might reveal the necessity for a change in staffing patterns to offer more comprehensive services at home. The results of this type of group study could be utilized as a program evaluation measurement for adequacy, effectiveness, efficiency, and appropriateness. The effectiveness of teaching a therapeutic home care program to clients with chronic obstructive pulmonary disease could be assessed according to the evidence of changes in client behavior and compliance. The findings may show that a different approach should be tried. Basic to this may be the need for more inservice education for the staff, including the emotional aspects of this disease.

PSROs

Professional Standards Review Organizations, or PSROs, as they are more commonly called, were mandated by law through the Social Security Act (as amended), Section 1115 (g), C42 USC, Section 1320 C-4 (g). These organizations are responsible for assessing the health care that Medicare and Medicaid clients receive to make sure that the services are medically necessary, appropriate, and of the highest quality. Initially, the focus of the program was on the care received in a hospital, but it has now expanded to include long-term care facilities. Home health agencies are not involved in the PSRO program at present, but undoubtedly they will be in the near future. To prepare for this, some agencies have already initiated internal peer review systems. As an example, the Community Health Nursing division of the Multnomah County Division of Health Services in Portland, Oregon, has implemented a program to review peers' working relationships and leadership potential (Johnson and Zimmerman 1975, pp. 618–619). The results of this review are used in conjunction with supervisory and self-evaluations to determine salary increments and promotion. Constructive relationships are a necessary part of the nursing process; to have a workable team approach, there must be interaction within the system. This example is just one small facet in peer review—this will have to extend to other areas and other professionals in the home health care system.

Problem-Oriented Record System

In many agencies, the problem-oriented record system has become an accepted and preferred method of encouraging more individualized case management. This system entails comprehensive data collection, problem identification, care plans pertaining to active problems, and continuing reevaluation of the client status and problem solution. A data base is established with information about the client's medical diagnosis or symptomatology, present physical and emotional condition, past history, and socioeconomic status. Client problems (physical, emotional, social, economic) are identified, and then goals and care plans are developed that relate to problem solution. These plans include collection of incomplete data, case management, and client education. Narrative notes are written in a SOAP format so that a specific problem is discussed according to Subjective (what the client or others say), Objective (what the professional observes or measures), Assessment (what this may mean), and Plan (what they will do about it). This procedure reduces long, wordy charting that often does not show relationships among the findings and yet is time-consuming for the writer as well as the reader. This system leads to more specific recording, aimed toward looking for relationships and meanings. The problem-oriented method lends itself readily to the audit process and to the evaluation of intervention and outcome. Coordination and communication among the disciplines pertaining to client care are improved. It is a systematic approach to client management with the goal of improving quality of care.

Need for Change

It is imperative that criteria, tools, type of data collected, research findings, and other quality assurance components be disseminated and shared in the health care system. Without uniform statistical reporting, no valid comparisons can be made among home health agencies at present. One of the recognized disease classification systems needs to be used by all agencies. The expertise of medical records specialists should be utilized to improve the system of record-keeping, data collection, and statistical reporting. There are wide variations in costs for home health services; better accounting systems and cost controls are vital. Support services to reduce the clerical duties of professional staffs must be encouraged. For example, routine reviews of client records is often a supervisory function, but this could better be performed by a trained medical records clerk using a deficiency checklist. The supervisor could use this time more advantageously to make quality audits or reviews and have conferences with the staff to improve client care. Variations in policies on admissions, discharges, length of stay, and number of visits according to condition demonstrate the need for established guidelines. If the personnel within the system do not develop the necessary criteria for accountability, the third-party reimbursers will continue to make the rules. These often seem arbitrary, inappropriate for the clients' well-being, and punitive toward the providers. The lack of courses on fiscal management in nursing education must be rectified. Effective and knowledgeable nurse-administrators are needed in the increasingly complex home health field. Community health care is expanding rapidly and will become an even larger part of the total health care delivery system. Therefore, those in this field need to work closely in order to identify strengths and weaknesses, problems and solutions.

Current nurse practice legislation in many states is recognizing the independent functions of nursing. However, with recognition comes increased responsibility and liability. Within and without the profession, a considerable effort has been made to define and evaluate the practice of nursing. As the momentum grows, techniques of evaluation will become more sophisticated and scientific. The individual practitioner, the organization, and funding sources can all profit a great deal from improved methods of evaluation and from seeking excellence in the performance and delivery of health care services. Ultimately, it is the consumer who will benefit from carefully planned, implemented, and evaluated professional care.

SUMMARY

Evaluation of a health system requires many types of review, from appraisal of the whole system to that of any individual member of the system. The objectives are to identify unmet needs and improve services in the most cost-effective way. (See Chapter 9 for a discussion of the cost-effectiveness of home health care versus hospitalization.) Adequacy, appropriateness, efficiency, and effectiveness are examined by means of a systematic and continuous study of the organization and its elements within the total environment. The results are measured according to their ability to promote internal and external change.

REFERENCES

Berkoben, Rita M. 1976, *Quality assurance in home health care*. Camp Hill, Pa.: Pennsylvania Assembly of Home Health Agencies.

Conditions of participation. 1974. Home Health Agencies Regulation No. 5. Federal Health Insurance for the Aged, HEW, SSA Subpart L. Rev 18. Washington, D.C.: Government Printing Office (9–74): 405–1229.

Feitelberg, Samuel B. 1975. *The problem oriented record system in physical therapy*. Burlington, Vermont.: University of Vermont Medical Center.

Freeman, Ruth; and Holmes, Edward. 1960. *Administration of public health services*. Philadelphia: Saunders.

Guidelines for utilization of specialized rehabilitation services in home health agencies. 1978. Task Force of the Home Health Agency Assembly of New Jersey, Inc., Princeton, N.J.: Home Health Agencies Assembly of New Jersey.

Harnish, Yvonne. 1976. *Patient care guides*. National League for Nursing Publication No. 21-1610. New York.

Johnson, Karen J.; and Zimmerman, Mary Ann. 1975. Peer review in a health department. *American Journal of Nursing* 75,4:618–619.

Kleffel, Dorothy. 1972. *A utilization review program for home health agencies*. Department of Health, Education and Welfare Publication No. HSM 72-6502. Washington, D.C.: U.S. Govt. Printing Office.

———, and Wilson, Elizabeth. 1976. *Evaluation handbook for home health programs*. Department of Health, Education and Welfare Publication No. HSA 76-3003. Washington, D.C.; U.S. Govt. Printing Office.

Lindeman, Carol. 1976. Measuring quality of nursing care, Part I. *Journal of Nursing Administration* 6,5:7–9.

———. 1976. Measuring quality of nursing care, Part II. *Journal of Nursing Administration* 6,3:16–19.

National League for Nursing. 1976. *Accreditation of home health agencies and community nursing services*. Council of Home Health Agencies and Community Health Services Publication No. 21-1306. New York.

———. 1973. *Utilization review—some directions*. Committee to Study Utilization Review Processes. New York: Council of Home Health Agencies and Community Health Services.

Phaneuf, Maria C. 1972. *The nursing audit—profile for excellence*. New York: Appleton-Century-Crofts.

Rotkovich, Rachel. 1976. The heartbeat of nursing services. Standard IV. *Journal of Nursing Administration* 6,4: 32–35.

Schell, P.; and Campbell, A. 1972. POMR—Not just another way to chart. *Nursing Outlook* 20,8:510–514.

Watson, A.; and Mayers, M. 1976. Evaluating the quality of patient care through retrospective chart review. *Journal of Nursing Administration* 6,3:17–21.

Weinstein, Edwin L. 1976. Developing a measure of the quality of nursing care. *Journal of Nursing Administration* 6,6:1–3.

Part Two

Nursing Alternatives within the System

This section presents the role of the nurse-manager as a change agent in different organizational settings. Health care organizations are struggling to adapt to many demands made by an environmental system that is rapidly changing. The ensuing stress overload can have a positive value in providing motivation for change among dissatisfied subsystems. Nurse-managers are in a position to be able to diagnose organizational problems, develop new adaptive mechanisms, and reduce tension.

In initiating change, the nurse-manager must choose a target system—the organization structure, the work itself, or the people who do the work. The next step is to recognize that change occurs as a process over time. Kurt Lewin has described a three-phase model of change:

Phase I. Unfreezing means "disturbing the peace" or upsetting the equilibrium of a system so that individuals or groups become aware of their discomfort and seek a change. Points of stress and strain in a system are stimulants for change.

Phase II. Moving to a new level is the action of changing itself. The changed system becomes more comfortable as barriers to changing are removed, or motivating forces are increased. Individuals or groups look to important people to validate their "new" selves.

Phase III. Refreezing occurs when new beliefs, actions or attitudes are perceived to be comfortable, and important others reinforce the change. A stable pattern of the changed behavior indicates that a relatively permanent, new state of equilibrium has been reached.

Resistance to change as an inevitable reality has to be dealt with by the change agent. Analyzing the modes of resistance and developing methods to deal with it are a major concern for the authors who discuss changing the organizational environment through the management process.

Chapter 6 describes the development of an autonomous group as a viable means for nurses to govern and control their own activities. Having learned collaborative skills in their peer groups, nurses can employ communication strategies to develop relationships of mutual interest and respect with other health care professionals. Autonomy and collaboration as concepts set the tone for the following chapters.

Chapter 7 explains assertiveness as a basic strategy that nurses need to become effective managers. Examples and exercises are suggested to give practice in assertive behavior.

Chapter 8 defines hospitalization as a dehumanizing experience and discusses the factors that contribute to dehumanized nursing care. Team nursing and primary nursing are compared in terms of giving client and nurse satisfaction. It is suggested that primary care is an organizational system of nursing that humanizes care.

Chapter 9 describes the role of the clinical nurse specialist as an agent of change. Examples demonstrate successful implementation of the role, as well as several instances of difficulty due to the organization structure, ambiguity in the role, and lack of support systems.

Chapter 10 discusses the role of the head nurse, including the dilemmas of inadequate preparation, the dual role of nurse and manager, and the necessity of interacting with many subsystems. Decision-making styles, communication, and relationships are the major tools used by the head nurse to turn organization goals into concrete actions.

Chapter 11 suggests that performance contracting is one way that nurse-managers can make objectives and standards explicit, thereby reducing tension between the nurse-manager and staff member. A participative objective-setting process is described in six steps for writing a contract.

Chapter 12 explains client advocacy as the action of defending or intervening on behalf or in the interest of the client. Nurses are clients' advocates when they uphold the clients' rights to participate in decision-making about their health care. The advantages and disadvantages of the role are mentioned.

Chapter 13 documents the case for noninstitutional care in favor of the services of a home health agency. Strategies for intervening in the larger systems that affect health care delivery are analyzed.

Chapter 14 describes the legislative process and political workings that pertain to nurses who want to influence health care services. Factors that affect nurses' political activism are explored, as well as the effects of nurse practice acts.

Chapter 15 shows a nurse utilizing political methods to achieve change as a colleague in an HSA. The National Health Planning and Resources Development Act is explained as it relates to the development and operation of a Health Systems Agency.

Chapter 16 is an action research study that describes why this method of research is appropriate for nurses, and how it was used with nurses on a collaborative project. The five phases of the action research process are presented, with examples taken from the researcher's perspective.

Chapter 17 gives the viewpoint of the action research group. The chapter also presents the functions of a working committee using participative management.

Chapter 18 goes beyond participative management to self-management, that is, control of the work situation by those who are doing the work. The historical development of this movement here and abroad is noted, and ways to institute self-management in health care systems are listed. The role of unions is also mentioned.

Chapter 19 discusses management in health care centers that fulfill the needs of specific communities, outside the traditional agencies. Issues of overlapping roles, the burnout phenomenon, responsiveness to community needs, and intra- and extraagency coordination are spelled out as unique aspects of this management system.

Chapter 20 describes the teaching-learning process as it affects education for leadership. Faculty and student roles are examined as they exist today, and suggestions are made for encouraging teachers and students to take responsibility for using learning experiences in leadership as a vehicle for change.

Chapter 6

Considerations in Developing Alternatives: Autonomy and Collaboration

Carole A. Shea and Carolyn Chambers Clark

OBJECTIVES

After studying this chapter, the learner will:

- Define autonomy in professional nursing
- Describe ways to become autonomous
- Define collaboration as a communication process
- Identify conditions that promote collaboration

CHANGING HEALTH CARE SYSTEM

In a rapidly changing health care system, nurses are finding that reliance on familar stereotypes, traditional policies and procedures, and outdated relationship patterns hinder their development as effective practitioners. There are many reasons for changes in the system, including basic preparation at the baccalaureate level for nurses, the "reality shock" encountered by new graduates, expanded roles that reflect clinical competence and leadership abilities, client advocacy and clients' rights, cost-effectiveness analysis of health care delivery, new organizational structures that use primary care nursing, and the increased use of multidisciplinary teams. Nurses are given the tools necessary for practice—theoretical knowledge and clinical skills—through their higher education. However, this is not sufficient preparation for working in the environment of complex organizations. Interaction with members of many subsystems, utilization of increasingly complicated technologies, and the expanded roles for professionals require a reordering of the division of labor. For nurses to function effectively and receive satisfaction from their work, they must develop new skills. Nurses must learn to tolerate ambiguity and to accept change as inevitable, ongoing, and increasing. Ways to cope with change include planning for it, recognizing and handling conflict (see Chapter 3), developing an autonomous group that defines professional identity and learns how to assume power and exert influence, and establishing collaborative relationships with other professionals. This chapter discusses autonomy and collaboration as they affect nurses.

DEFINITION OF AUTONOMY

Being autonomous means being self-governing. Individual nurses act autonomously when they act spontaneously, deciding what action to take, and choosing a purposeful direction. When they consciously, not compulsively, make decisions, they have freedom to practice nursing. Autonomy and self-actualization is the highest developmental level of the healthy, mature person (Grissum and Spengler 1976, pp. 68–69).

Professional autonomy in nursing means that nurses govern and control their own activities. Nurse practitioners collectively determine and regulate the management of their profession, while practitioners individually maintain control of and are accountable for their own clinical judgments and practices.

Autonomy is granted to professional workers because of their particular knowledge. Since the knowledge is specialized, only members of that profession are deemed competent to define necessary and safe practice. However, it is not unusual for human beings to become more concerned with their own functions or the existence of their own systems. Therefore, professionals must demonstrate accountability for their actions and commitment to the use of their special knowledge on the client's behalf (Maas and Jacox 1977, pp. 17–19). Thus, autonomy is directly tied to accountability and client advocacy.

Hierarchical and bureaucratic organization is incompatible with professional autonomy for nurses. In bureaucratic organizations nurses are often viewed as semiprofessionals with less knowledge than "full" professionals such as doctors. For this reason, nurses have less autonomy and are more subject to control by the administrative hierarchy than other professionals in the same system. In such systems, physician control is fostered by legal and administrative regulations which restrict nurses' access to clients, to third-party payments, and to the consultative services or referral of clients to and from other experts. As some nurses become more automonous and seek fewer administrative controls over their practice, there will undoubtedly be role strains and resistance to these changes. Nurses who are comfortable in the semiprofessional role, and physicians and others who have authority will exert pressure on autonomy-seeking nurses either to cease their efforts or to accept less autonomy than they want. In systems terms, this can be viewed as an attempt to maintain the steady state or reestablish equilibrium. If autonomy is achieved, change and adaptation will occur through positive feedback. If autonomy is not achieved, the status quo will be maintained.

Maas and Jacox (1977, pp. 24–29) contend that there are four prerequisites to nurse autonomy. One is direct access to clients without the physician's order. Another is decentralization of the nursing hierarchy with primary nursing care and 24-hour, 7-days-a-week accountability for clients. A third prerequisite is peer evaluation and supervision of practice; this means that only nurses evaluate and supervise one another's practice. A final condition is the formation of a cohesive group of professional colleagues or peers. Such a group enables nurses to define standards of practice and to regulate practice through peer evaluation and supervision.

Once a group of nurses can work together in an open system that allows change, the dimensions of autonomy can be developed and defined. Such dimensions include identification of the areas of health care to which professional nurses lay claim, the expected outcomes of nurse and client behavior that will be used to measure acceptable nursing practice, the structure and function of the nursing system, qualifications required for those who practice nursing, and the dissemination and discovery of knowledge. Autonomous nurses assume that the requirements of client accountability can be met by measuring individual practice against specified standards, designing a systematic method to determine the effectiveness of the nursing care delivery system, providing clinical consultation to peers, interviewing potential professional nurses, and validating and applying nursing theory and knowledge (Maas and Jacox 1977, pp. 24–27).

THE ROAD TO AUTONOMY

As a predominantly female group, nurses are influenced by social expectations. Women are trained to be unsure of goals, to wait to see what is available, or to be told what to do. Women often come to nursing with the mental injunction "Don't think." Thinking and deciding what is needed or wanted is the first step in taking power (Wyckoff 1977, p. 71). As products of our culture, nurses are not sure how to take assertive, autonomous action. For this reason (as well as the "power in numbers" rationale) nurses need to form a cohesive, supportive peer group. The group's reassurance is vital in the process of raising one's self-esteem and self-confidence. In forming such a group, there should be one or more nurses who are experienced in group processes and group leadership; their participation can encourage feedback. When both group task and maintenance functions have been fulfilled, cohesiveness develops, and the group can attain its goals by means of positive feedback. If either the task or maintenance functions are not fulfilled, the status quo is maintained and autonomy cannot be achieved (as a result of negative feedback).

The group can promote individual and group autonomy by not allowing its members to take helpless or rescuer roles (Wyckoff 1977, pp. 90–100); all members are expected to be competent and working participants. This message is communicated both verbally and nonverbally. Rescuing reinforces passivity and helplessness. Group autonomy cannot be achieved if group members communicate the following message to one another: "Let me help you; you can't do it, but I can." In an autonomous group the members accept each other as they are at the moment, recognizing their limitations and their potentialities. Adopting the rescuer role—giving more than one gets, rather than insisting that all members of the group perform and take equal responsibility—leads to attempts to blame the participants of the subsystem or the system, rather than to move toward autonomy. Part of learning how to form a cohesive nursing group is learning how to set limits with one another. Nurses frequently have difficulty saying "no." Unless this limitation is worked through, illegitimate requests or criticisms can paralyze the group process and limit autonomy.

Argyris (1977, p. 123) has identified a number of power dilemmas that pertain to nurses who want to form autonomous groups. These dilemmas are perhaps best posed as questions.

1   How can strength and power be promoted while recognizing the dilemmas and inconsistencies of health care systems?

2   How can group members behave openly and directly without controlling others?

3   How can the nursing group be advocates of its own views and still encourage confrontation and disagreement or divergent views?

4   How can individual nurses within the group decrease their own anxiety about their actions in order to respond effectively to others' fears and anxieties?

5   How can the nursing group gain credibility when its members may be uncomfortable or unsure of its actions?

Claus and Bailey (1977, pp. 91–172) discuss various ways nurses can develop power and influence, including:

1   Build a positive self-concept and high self-esteem by praising oneself and others, by setting realistic goals, and by evaluating oneself realistically—comparing one's initial behaviors with present behaviors.
2   Build a climate of trust by focusing on *what* happened, and not who did it.
3   Equalize the amount of feedback expected from others with self-disclosure (sharing of feelings about events using "I" statements, such as "I feel . . . ").
4   Develop specific goals that are measurable and attainable.
5   Practice clear and effective communication.
6   Set up ongoing work groups where communication lines are open, leadership is shared, procedures are developed to guide action, and problem-solving processes are used.

The road to autonomy requires a commitment on the part of individual nurses to meet regularly and purposely to chisel out issues and decide on appropriate action. It also means that the director of nursing should share decision making with the group. Participative management enables nurses to use their special knowledge in concert with others. It also teaches nurses how to manage and conveys the following: "You are important," "You can decide," "You have an obligation to participate," and "You are not helpless or impotent."

It may be that the nursing group will have to form a bargaining unit with the state nurses association in order to establish formal negotiations with agency administrators (Maas and Jacox 1977, p. 49). To risk the possible censure that may result, nurses must act together. Although nurses are loathe to use medicine as a role model (and certainly there have been many instances of negative modeling), when a doctor takes a stand or is attacked, the medical association tends to close ranks and deflect the attack. When a nurse takes a stand for which he or she is attacked, other nurses frequently turn their backs or sigh, "Thank God, it wasn't me!" If the group decided to take a stand, the responsibility for doing so would more likely be shared since there would be greater commitment. Of course, nurses need practice in learning how to participate in management. The first step, however, seems to be nurses' recognition of their inherent power both individually and collectively.

DEFINITION OF COLLABORATION

As nurses develop an autonomous group, they learn how to collaborate as colleagues. They come to value and respect their peers who share a mutual interest in providing quality health care. Once intraprofessional collaboration has been established, nurses can attempt to become colleagues of other health care professionals, principally physicians.

Collaboration is primarily a communication process that occurs when persons of different skills work together as a team to achieve a specified goal. Collaboration is the interactive relationship among individuals who share the same goals, philosophy, and purpose; who understand each other's professional and personal skills; and who value each other's unique characteristics (Aradine 1973, p. 656). Collaboration is a joint problem-solving process that requires maturity, openness, sensitivity, adaptability, and trust. There is a need for feedback to enhance positive results and to eliminate negative factors that would prevent adequate functioning.

Cohen (1973, p. 244) states that "people and systems seem to work best when the collaboration serves the interest of each, and when each has a distinctly different but complementary role to play in the total endeavor." Sharp demarcations and boundaries between professional roles are not as evident in health care systems as they once were. Expanding roles, changing delivery patterns, consumerism, and the development of new technologies lead to overlapping functions and areas of expertise held in common by professionals of different backgrounds and education. The blurring of professional roles often leads to incompatibility and conflict rather than complementarity and collaboration.

DIFFICULTIES IN COLLABORATION

Conflict is generated when work assignments require negotiation because two or more persons from different backgrounds can perform the same job equally well (Smoyak 1977, p. 54). Resolution of who does what to whom and when will depend upon the situation—who is available, what the organizational environment is, how much time is required, and the type of client. Nurses and physicians may perform the same tasks in some instances, or, because of their different education and professional perspective, they may work in concert using different skills.

Collaboration often takes place in the context of consultation and referral among colleagues. Physicians are trained to seek, offer, and provide assistance by consultation. However, while some nurses do consult and collaborate with one another, most nurses do not relate to other nurses as peers. Instead, their behavior reflects a superior-subordinate relationship (Munn 1977, pp. 100–101). Some factors that hinder nurses' use of consultation and referral include their subordinate self-image, the status of women in our society, a diploma-school heritage of servitude, the bureaucratic hierarchy of organizations, their personality traits, and the lack of rewards for nurse colleagueship (Nolan 1976, p. 43). Physicians successfully use consultation and referral because their education fosters it, and these practices guard their professional freedom by allowing physicians to refuse to become involved, or to be able to negotiate how the collaboration will take place (Bergen 1965, p. 1064). Collaboration entails some loss of autonomy. For nurses, collaboration with physicians is a double-edged sword; they may have to relinquish some newly won autonomy for egalitarian status as colleagues. Formerly, nurses did not speak the same language as physicians because of their lack of academic preparation, and their different social background, economic status, and career aspirations. Now with an emphasis on baccalaureate preparation, more adequate compensation, less disparity in social class, and the greater career orientation of nurses, communication among all professionals is facilitated. Of course, the nurse is not the only one who must cope with the loss of familiar roles and changing expectations. The physician must also learn to adapt to change; they are not immune to fear, a sense of loss, territoriality, competition, helplessness, powerlessness, and anxiety that cause them to fall back on the familiar rigid roles and close disciplinary circles. However, clients with health care needs are not a scarce commodity engendering competition. Collaboration (rather than competition) is a rational strategy that can benefit all professionals.

COLLABORATION AT WORK

Nurses, physicians, and other providers of health care collaborate most effectively under the following conditions (Smoyak 1977, p. 57):

1 Mutual agreement on a goal.
2 Equality in status and personal interactions.
3 A shared base of scientific and professional knowledge with complementary diversity in skills, expertise, and practices.
4 Mutual trust and respect for each other's competence.

Interprofessional collaboration occurs in phases (Jacobson 1974, pp. 751–755); initially there is an enthusiastic, open interest in others' abilities, and communication is directed toward finding out "Who are you professionally?" This is followed by self-disclosure and the building of mutual trust through discovery. Insecurity develops as a struggle against closeness emerges. This is followed by a tug of war that is exemplified by defending professional values, protecting territory, and asserting who is right and who is wrong. At this stage the focus is on manifest differences between the professions. This may degenerate into personal attacks on individuals according to built-in prejudices and stereotypes, leading to mistrust, rejection, insulation, and withdrawal. Groups that survive this hostility reaffirm their purpose once the biases are made known. Finally, there is an identification with others, emphasizing the commonness of purpose and strengthening the professional identities, which is facilitated by verbal and nonverbal communication.

Nurses participating in a collaborative project need to demonstrate a congruence between their beliefs and their behavior. Through reality-based self-esteem, collective assurance, and a strong professional identity, nurses can communicate that they *know* what they know. They must act on the knowledge that their professional skills are a valued resource. An open dialogue indicating a willingness to listen as well as to share ideas will help to change attitudinal sets.

Nurses can learn to collaborate as they work with other professionals on research projects, in seminar workshops, as members of interdisciplinary health care teams, and as consultants in the community. It would be helpful if nursing students could learn how to work collaboratively during their educational preparation by sharing clinical experiences, didactic presentations, and discussion seminars with other students from medicine, social work, and psychology. Admittedly, it might be difficult to inculcate a strong professional identity if nursing students have the opportunity to understand and empathize with the diverse value systems, goals, and needs of other disciplines (Sifneos 1968, pp. 124–125). Research needs to be done to identify the characteristics of collaboration and to develop methods for promoting interprofessional collaboration.

The Surgeon General's Report on Extending the Scope of Nursing Practice (1971, p. 7) concluded that:

> A redefinition of the functional interaction of medicine and nursing is essential . . . in terms of their respective roles in the provision of health services rather than in terms of professional boundaries and rigid lines of responsibility.

As nurses' roles become expanded, competitive feelings, professional jealousies, antagonisms, misunderstandings, and ambiguous lines of authority make meaningful communcation difficult. If individuals are not to become incapacitated by role strain and frustration, the health care organization must foster interprofessional communication and provide a structure and environment that facilitate change. Nurses as a group stand to benefit from collaborative interactions; therefore, they must take an active part in making the necessary changes in the health care organization.

SUMMARY

Nurses who want to develop alternatives that foster independent nursing practice must become autonomous and learn to collaborate with other professionals. Autonomy means acting in such a way that nurses control and govern their own activities. Nurses are granted autonomy because they possess special knowledge. Autonomy is directly tied to accountability and client advocacy. Autonomy is developed and defined by nurses who work together as a cohesive unit in an open system. As an autonomous group, nurses can gain power and influence.

Once nurses learn to interact as professional colleagues, they can begin to collaborate effectively with other professionals. Collaboration is a communication process between persons who share goals, understand each other's skills, and value each other's unique characteristics. People collaborate best when the project serves the interest of each, and each has a different but complementary role to play. Nurses and physicians have difficulty establishing a collaborative relationship when their roles are blurred, their skills are similar, authority lines are unclear, and different educational backgrounds and social lifestyles prevent them from speaking the same language. Nurses can develop collaborative skills by recognizing the phases of collaboration; projecting a competent, knowledgeable self-image; and by promoting an open dialogue to change attitudes and practices. It is suggested that nursing students be educated to value and use the collaborative process by sharing clinical experiences, class work, and discussion with their peers and students in other disciplines.

REFERENCES

Aradine, Carolyn R.; and Pridham, Karen F. 1973. Model for collaboration. *Nursing Outlook* 21,10:655–657.

Argyris, Chris. 1977. Double loop learning in organization. *Harvard Business Review* 55,5:115–125.

Bergen, Bernard J. 1965. Professional communities and the evaluation of demonstration projects in community mental hospitals. *American Journal of Public Health* 55,7:1057–1066.

Claus, Karen E.; and Bailey, June T. 1977. *Power and influence in health care.* St. Louis: Mosby.

Cohen, Raquel E. 1973. The collaborative coprofessional: developing a new mental health role. *Hospital and Community Psychiatry* 24,4:242–245.

Grissum, Marlene; and Spengler, Carol. 1976. *Womenpower and health care.* Boston: Little, Brown.

Jacobson, Sylvia. 1974. A study of interprofessional collaboration. *Nursing Outlook* 22,12:751–755.

Maas, Meridean; and Jacox, Ada K. 1977. *Guidelines for nurse autonomy/patient welfare.* New York: Appleton-Century-Crofts.

Munn, Yvonne L. 1977. Power: how to get and use it in nursing today. *Nursing Administrative Quarterly* 1,1:95–103.

Nolan, Mary Gill. 1976. Wanted: colleagueship in nursing. *Journal of Nursing Administration* 6,2:41–43.

Sifneos, Peter E. 1969. The interdisciplinary team. *Psychiatric Quarterly* 43:123–130.

Smoyak, Shirley A. 1977. Problems in interprofessional relations. *Bulletin of New York Academy of Medicine* 53,1:51–59.

Surgeon general's report: extending the scope of nursing practice. 1971. Washington, D.C.: U.S. Govt. Printing Office.

Wyckoff, Hogie. 1977. *Solving women's problems.* New York: Grove Press.

Chapter 7

Assertiveness Training as Preparation

Carolyn Chambers Clark

OBJECTIVES

After studying this chapter, the learner will:

- Define assertiveness in nursing
- Differentiate between assertive and aggressive behavior
- List five areas where nurses can become more assertive
- List five ways nurses can practice to become more assertive

ASSERTIVENESS DEFINED

Assertiveness includes aspects of freedom and control, rights, obligations, responsibility, respect and activity, and communication. The freedom aspect of assertiveness is the freedom for nurses to reveal themselves through words and actions. An assertive person demonstrates through words and actions: "This is me. This is what I think. This is what I feel. This is what I want."

The control element of assertiveness in nursing is the nurses' realization that they have control over what happens to them, that they can make choices about when and how to use that control, and that they cannot control others' behavior, only their own.

Nurses are joining the list of groups who are beginning to define their rights as people, including mental patients, consumers, and women. Smith (1975, pp. 24–74) presents the following "Bill of Assertive Rights":

1   You have the right to judge your own behavior, thoughts, and emotions, and to take the responsibility for their initiation and consequences upon yourself.

2   You have the right to offer no reasons or excuses to justify your behavior.

3   You have the right to judge if you are responsible for finding solutions to other people's problems.

4   You have the right to change your mind.

5   You have the right to make mistakes—and be responsible for them.

6   You have the right to say, "I don't know."

7   You have the right to be independent of the goodwill of others before coping with them.

8   You have the right to be illogical in making decisions.

9   You have the right to say, "I don't understand."

10   You have the right to say, "I don't care."

11   You have the right to say "no" and not feel guilty.

Fensterheim (1975, p. 49) has drawn up a different set of assertive rights:

1   You have the right to do anything so long as it does not hurt someone else.

2   You have the right to maintain your dignity by being properly assertive—even if it hurts someone else—as long as your motive is assertive and not aggressive.

3   You always have the right to make a request of another person as long as you realize the other person has the right to say "no."

4   You must realize that there are certain borderline cases in interpersonal situations where rights aren't clear. But you always have the right to discuss the problem with the other person in order to clarify it.

5   You have the right to attain your rights!

Fagin (1975, p. 84) has listed the following nurses' rights:

1   The right to find dignity in self-expression and self-enhancement by using our special abilities and educational background.

2   The right to recognition for our contribution by means of an environment in which we can practice, and receive proper, professional economic rewards.

3 The right to a work environment that will minimize physical and emotional stress and health risks.

4 The right to control what is professional practice within the limits of the law.

5 The right to set standards for excellence in nursing.

6 The right to participate in policy-making that affects nursing.

7 The right to social and political action on behalf of nursing and health care.

As with any set of rights, the chooser may decide to exercise all or some of them. Once the nurse knows the limits of control and acts on any of these rights, a set of responsibilities follows; the major one is responsibility for one's own action. By becoming assertive, nurses risk the consequences of their statements and actions. Daring to assert one's rights can be a heady, if anxiety-provoking experience. Any change the nurse begins to take will no doubt lead to certain feelings of anxiety and unsureness. With practice, however, assertive behavior can become part of any nurse's style of relating.

Being assertive also carries with it certain respect, for example, the enhancement of one's own self-respect. The assertive nurse is aware that he or she cannot always win or be right. Part of being assertive is the need to know and accept one's own limitations and strengths. The assertive person also has an active orientation to life. In contrast to the passive person, who sits back and waits for things to happen, the assertive person sets goals and works toward them in order to influence the future.

In order to be assertive, the nurse must communicate clearly and consistently. Nurses must convey messages to others about their wishes, needs, intentions, knowledge, or practice. For example, if a nurse says smilingly and meekly to a physician, "No, I can't do that now; I'm talking with a patient," but then agrees to help the doctor if he or she asks again, no clear, consistent message has been given. Rather, the nurse has conveyed several conflicting messages about his or her intention and practice.

Essentially, *assertiveness in nursing* is: setting goals, acting on those goals in a clear and consistent manner, and taking responsibility for the consequences of one's actions.

ASSERTIVE VERSUS AGGRESSIVE BEHAVIOR

Aggressive behavior differs from assertive behavior mainly in that the former attempts to control or manipulate another person (even though it may be subtle). Aggressive behavior can be passive, for example, the nurse who always "forgets" to bring a verbally angry patient his medication, or the nursing administrator who is chronically late for appointments with the staff. Other examples of hidden aggression include: sharing confidential information with the staff in order to embarrass the one who has confided, procrastinating, being overly helpful and thus stifling another person's independence, nagging, developing physical symptoms, wishing to escape from the issue, inducing guilt in another person, criticizing unfairly, and teasing.

Whatever the form of hidden aggression, it is clear that the person feels uncomfortable about making a clear statement of his or her feelings; therefore, he or she uses devious and unclear methods to express anger. The results are usually frustrating; more resentment and anger occur on both sides, while the real issue is submerged.

Assertive training would allow the nurse to break the cycle of resentment, anger, or anxiety by learning how to communicate clearly to others without feeling belittled, unloved, or rejected. It is impossible to be an effective nurse-manager if one is overwhelmed by others' behavior; being overwhelmed leads to avoidance or overly aggressive behavior.

Active aggression is a direct maneuver to control another person, but this may becloud the issue. For example, a supervisor may be able to intimidate a head nurse or student by yelling at them, although the issue may not be anger. Or, a patient can hit a nurse and actively show anger when actually he may be angry with his mother. Active aggression may be easier for some people to handle because it is more readily identifiable. Passive aggression may be more difficult to deal with because it may not be recognized; nurses may not realize that they have been the target of another's hidden aggression at the moment it occurs.

Assertive behavior differs from aggressive behavior in another important way. When people behave aggressively, they "come on too strong," or, in the case of passive aggression, "too deviously" or unclearly. While aggressive behavior may help to achieve goals temporarily, most of the time communication is disrupted, and others may counterattack with active or passive aggression. In contrast, assertive behavior does not guarantee goal achievement, but it can lead to an increased sense of self-esteem and well-being. When an assertive person does not reach a goal, he or she is temporarily disappointed, but not irrationally hostile. Besides, since the assertive person has an active orientation toward life, he or she is likely to try again because of the knowledge that things do not always happen as desired.

INHIBITORY FACTORS

It seems fairly simple to know what one's rights, responsibilities, and obligations are, and to stand up for them. In practice, however, there are many reasons why nurses find assertive behavior difficult, including socialization practices, nursing education, and health care systems norms.

Socialization

Since nurses have for the most part been socialized into the female role, they may find it particularly difficult to be assertive because they fear any or all of the following: being rejected; being "unfeminine"; being "aggressive"; being confronted; losing such protective measures as blaming others; losing control of oneself in crying, yelling, or screaming (basically this is a fear of confronting one's own anger); learning the truth about oneself; being retaliated against; or being punished by authority figures.

Nursing Education

Although nurse educators are beginning to prepare students to develop many more nursing skills, there has been little attempt, if any, to teach novices how to assert themselves as skilled practitioners. In fact, nursing instructors may be helping to keep nurses "down" by treating students as inept children who must be watched as they draw up medications; and by stepping in to handle conflicts between head nurses and students, between students and doctors, and between clients and students.

Of course, some nurse educators believe that students can teach and supervise one another (Nehren 1968; Burnside 1971; C. Clark, 1976), but in general, they seem to be overprotective of students and overdefensive in their relationships with members of other professions. Perhaps this trend continues in nursing education because educators have not learned to be assertive themselves. Thus, nursing faculty tend to vacillate between submission (Stein 1968; Thomstad 1975) and attack toward physicians. For example, it is not uncommon to hear both undergraduate and graduate nursing faculties tell students about how they "got so mad at Doctor_____" that they either yelled out loud or withdrew in a huff to the coffee shop. With so few role models of assertive faculty members, nursing students cannot really be expected to practice assertive behavior simply by reading articles or books about independent nursing practice.

Some nurse educators may ask, "But doesn't assertiveness training teach nurses to be manipulative?" The answer is, "Yes, but all communication is an attempt to influence another person. In assertive stances, the nurse is clear and open about what is desired, whereas in aggressive stances, the nurse is unclear, devious, or irrational about what is desired."

Health Care Systems Norms

The norm in most health care systems is that the physician makes the decisions (despite written philosophies to the contrary). Because this is so, nurses who try to be assertive about their practice may meet negative reactions. For example, the nonassertive nursing group may side with the physican and exert pressure on the assertive nurse to submit and return to the flock. Trying to fight the tide of combined nurse-physician forces can be an extremely lonely and frustrating effort.

In many cases, the pressures from physicians are of less importance. Like any minority group, nurses face an antinurse prejudice from within their own ranks. Sometimes nurses are so ambivalent about their right to practice that they vacillate between talking with one another about one another and turning to one another for solace and support. However, their energies are now beginning to be directed toward more fruitful channels such as cooperative committee work and exerting political and economic pressure.

ASSERTIVENESS AND NURSING

There are quite a few areas in which more assertive behavior on the part of nurses can be an important asset in management. Nurses can learn to be more assertive in their relationships with students who are preparing for the nursing role, with those whom they supervise, with doctors, with nursing colleagues, with political leaders and legislators, and in their relationships with clients and their families. Assertive behavior can also be used to establish leadership and power in one-to-one relationships as well as in groups.

At this point, the reader might well ask, "But if you're a professional nurse, aren't you necessarily assertive?" The two are not coincident. In fact, as a profession, nurses seem to be afraid that it may be "impolite" or "unfeminine" or even "unprofessional" to assert their rights with peers, colleagues, or clients. Unfortunately, being "nice" takes its toll on the nurse, and resentment and anger are submerged and reappear as snide remarks, punitive tactics, blame-fixing, guilt-induction, and so on.

Changes Needed

Fensterheim (1975, p. 33) lists three levels of behavior that can be changed by means of assertiveness training. To become assertive, the nurse needs to make changes on all three levels. The first level, which is elementary and easily learned, includes making eye contact with others, standing or sitting straight, and speaking in a clear voice that can easily be heard. These simple nonverbal behaviors alone can make a difference in whether people pay attention to what the nurse says. Nurses who speak in rambling, monotonous, or barely audible voices, who look at the ceiling or floor, or who slouch or turn their bodies away from their audience are less likely to be listened to, despite the importance of their message.

The second level, which is verbal communication, includes saying "yes" when the nurse wishes to, and saying "no" when the nurse really does not wish to do something. Being able to ask for a favor and receive praise are also part of assertiveness. How to handle a "putdown" (without denying it, attacking the person who put one down, or sulking and then subtly retaliating) can be learned as well. Learning how to structure work time and other habits of daily living can also be included in this level.

The third level includes more complex interactions with people in the work setting and elsewhere. In general, though, being an assertive manager requires five basic skills:

1 An active orientation toward management, including thinking through work goals, the steps needed to achieve those goals, and deciding how a nurse can use his or her skills to best advantage.

2 The ability to do the job by learning better work habits, discipline, ability to concentrate, and setting limits on others' attempts to interfere or block goal attainment.

3 The ability to control anxieties and fears about how others will evaluate the nurse and his or her actions.

4 The ability to relate to peers, subordinates, and superiors in terms of cooperating, making requests, asking favors, taking compliments, handling putdowns, setting limits by saying "no" when appropriate, and structuring their activities.

5 The ability to negotiate the social system of the work setting; this means knowing what the norms for behavior are, where the resistance to change is greatest, how others have been successful in negotiating the system, and where the constraints are so great that change will probably not occur.

Thinking through Work Goals

Certainly the first, and perhaps the most important, change the manager needs to make in becoming assertive is to define the work goals and separate the irrational from the rational goals. The reality goals for the job may be very basic, for example, to earn a living; if this is the manager's chief goal, he or she had better acknowledge it in order to make subsequent decisions about the importance of working overtime and finding other sources of satisfaction outside work.

Another reality goal is to make as much money as possible. If this goal is chosen by the nurse-manager, he or she must be willing to sacrifice some leisure time, outside acitivities, and interpersonal relationships. Pressure, worries, and stress must also be accepted since it is not the *kind* of job that is important, but the opportunity for making money that will take precedence in this goal.

Still another reality goal is the pursuit of glory, status, or prestige. If this goal is chosen, the nurse-manager must be willing to take on the added responsibilities that go with status and prestige, as well as to deal with loneliness, since the higher one rises, the more others may attempt to undercut and undermine the manager's actions.

Yet another goal the manager might choose is to work where he or she will be rewarded for special interests and skills. If the manager achieves this position by default or seniority, there is little chance of attaining this goal; the manager can then decide to switch fields or learn new management skills.

Another goal the manager might choose is personal growth and change; if so, the manager must be ready to deal with subsequent challenges and the high levels of anxiety they may engender.

Finally, the manager may decide on the goal of doing socially meaningful work. Here, the implementation of a principle is the manager's reward. Whoever chooses this goal should be aware that few other people are motivated by this goal and should be prepared to devote many years to it, with very small increases in status, leisure, or money.

There are many unrealistic work goals that are likely to produce frustration for the manager who consciously or unconsciously chooses them. Some of these unrealistic goals are: the need to be needed, the need to be liked rather than respected, the need to master impossible situations, the need to be a "good child" by winning approval, and the need to have others feel sorry for you (Fensterheim 1975, pp. 253–254).

Assessing Assertiveness

In order for the nurse-manager to decide whether he or she needs to become more assertive, an assessment of assertiveness should be made. Table 7-1 lists some questions that will help the nurse-manager make such an assessment. Thus, the nurse-manager will be able to identify whether assertiveness training is needed in verbal and nonverbal presentation of self, in having an active orientation to the job, in structuring work habits, in controlling anxiety about others' evaluations, in relating to coworkers, or in being able to negotiate the system.

Setting Goals

If the nurse-manager needs to become more effective in setting goals, the following exercise is suggested. Take a piece of paper and divide it in half vertically with a pencil line. Then, fill in the information as given in Table 7-2. From this list of skills and goals, cross out those that are unrealistic or unrelated to what is asked for.

Table 7-1   Assertive Assessment

Answer the following statements either "yes" or "no." Total the "yeses" to determine how assertive you are.

Verbal and nonverbal style

_____	1	I always communicate what I want to communicate.
_____	2	I make frequent and direct eye contact with the other person when speaking.
_____	3	I speak loudly and firmly enough.
_____	4	I speak concisely and clearly.
• _____	5	I stick to the point I'm trying to make.
_____	6	I never apologize for the point I'm making.

TOTAL _____   Key: 6 = assertive; 4–5 nearly assertive; 3–0 need practice

Active orientation

_____	1	I like my work.
_____	2	I suggest new procedures, ideas, or theories.
_____	3	I work to my full capacity.
_____	4	I tell coworkers (teachers) what I expect from them.
_____	5	I ask coworkers (teachers) exactly what they expect from me.
_____	6	I work to make things turn out the way I want.

TOTAL _____   Key: 6 = assertive; 4–5 nearly assertive; 3–0 need practice

Work habits

_____	1	I structure my work day so that I am satisfied with its outcome.
_____	2	I tell others what the limits of their interruptions are.
_____	3	I can concentrate on one task at a time.
_____	4	I structure my work tasks so they can be completed on time.
_____	5	I structure my tasks so they can be completed with minimal stress.
_____	6	I structure my work to reward myself.

TOTAL _____   Key: 6 = assertive; 4–5 nearly assertive; 3–0 need practice

Control of anxiety and fear

_____	1	I can ask for a raise, promotion, or reasonable limit to my work load.
_____	2	I can limit personal chores for others I do not wish to do.
_____	3	I can arrive at work or school late or leave early occasionally without making excuses.
_____	4	I can confront an issue at work or school rather than calling in "sick."
_____	5	I can make legitimate requests from my boss or teacher without feeling guilty.
_____	6	I can take a compliment without getting flustered or denying it.
_____	7	I can listen to someone point out a mistake I've made without becoming upset.
_____	8	I can speak in a group without becoming uptight.
_____	9	I can tell others when I'm angry.
_____	10	I can give my viewpoint without qualifying my statements with comments such as, "I'm sorry to interrupt," "This is probably not right, but," or "This may be a dumb question to ask, but. . . ."
_____	11	I feel comfortable with authority figures.

Table 7-1   Assertive Assessment (continued)

_____	12	I don't fear being disliked.
_____	13	I can tolerate failure in myself.
_____	14	I can tolerate failure in others.
_____	15	I can deal with being ignored.
_____	16	I can stay "cool" when others scrutinize my work.
_____	17	I can deal with stress without getting tension headaches, diarrhea, etc.
_____	18	I can handle teasing by others.
_____	19	I can take a reasonable risk without fearing I'll fail or be fired.
TOTAL _____		Key: 19 = assertive; 15–18 nearly assertive; 14–0 need practice

Relating to coworkers

_____	1	I remind supervisees (clients, peers) of deadlines.
_____	2	I can handle putdowns without denying or overreacting to them.
_____	3	I can say "no" to others.
_____	4	I can deal with others' anger.
_____	5	I can work with others without nagging them.
_____	6	I can work with others without trying to make them feel guilty.
TOTAL _____		Key: 6 = assertive; 4–5 nearly assertive; 3–0 need practice

Negotiating the system

_____	1	I know what the norms and constraints of my job are.
_____	2	I feel comfortable negotiating my work system.
_____	3	I know how to introduce change effectively.
_____	4	I can speak to members of other disciplines as peers.
TOTAL _____		Key: 4 = assertive; 3 nearly assertive; 2–0 need practice

Table 7-2   Setting Work Goals

What kinds of management skills do I have?	What goals would I like to attain in the short range (this year)?
	In the long range (5–10 years hence)?

Changing Work Habits

Changing work habits requires a similar but somewhat different approach. Fensterheim has suggested the following three steps for identifying and changing a habit (1975, pp. 187–191). The first step is to identify the habit to be changed; this requires:

  1 Expressing the habit in behaviors that can be counted or measured. For example, to increase one's ability to concentrate on reports, the following behaviors could be counted: sitting at an office desk alone, taking no phone calls, allowing no one to enter the office.
  2 Counting the behaviors to see how often they occur now (count them for at least a week). This "before" phase will enable the nurse to check progress in changing the habit.
  3 Determining what precedes the habit behavior. For example, does the associate director of nursing always come in to chat, and this disrupts the ability to concentrate? Or, does the nurse start thinking about an unresolved argument or a pleasant weekend? Is there a beginning or midpoint where it would be possible to interrupt the habit? At what point does it seem possible to interrupt the habit?

  The second step is to make a contract of intention to change the habit; this can be done either with oneself or with someone else. The nurse has to make sure that the intention can actually be accomplished in the near future. The contract can be shown to someone who is in a position to monitor, but not nag or induce guilt about, the action. Select simple, easily attained goals. In the example above, a realistic contract might be: "I will spend one-half hour a week in my office alone looking at the report."
  The third step is to try to arrange the elements in the environment so that the desired behavior will be easy to attain. If the nurse is a head nurse, trying to concentrate on a report might be easy at 1:00 or 2:00 P.M., but not between 7:00 and 10:00 A.M. Try other ways to control stimuli that set off the undesired behavior, such as putting up a "Do Not Disturb" sign, locking an office door, or going to the hospital library.

PRACTICE IN BECOMING ASSERTIVE

Practicing to become more assertive is often begun more effectively outside the anxiety-provoking environment. The nurse-manager can use the following methods to practice assertiveness: attend assertiveness training workshops, practice written exercises, use tape-recorded exercises, do relaxation exercises, and use role playing/simulated situations.

Workshops

Various disciplines are beginning to offer workshops in assertive training. By contacting continuing education centers, the nurse-manager can keep abreast of what is available. Workshops usually provide a wide range of practice in assertive training; therefore, the nurse-manager who participates can gain valuable practical experience.

Written Exercises

Written exercises, such as the questionnaire in Table 7-1 and "Setting Work Goals" (Table 7-2), can help the nurse-manager focus on needed assertiveness skills.

Tape-Recorded Exercises

With the aid of a tape recorder, the nurse can practice elements of assertiveness that relate to clear communication. The tape recorder can be used in the following practice situations: asking for a promotion, speaking before a group, refusing a boss's request, accepting a compliment, reminding supervisees of deadlines, learning not to qualify statements, and handling putdowns. By visualizing the approximate situation, the nurse can turn the tape recorder on and record just what he or she plans to say in the actual situation. Then, the taped segment can be replayed and the nurse can evaluate whether the tone of voice sounds firm and whether the message sounds clear and consistent. A friend or colleague can also listen to the taped segment and make suggestions. Some situations, such as dealing with putdowns, might be handled by having a friend make putdown statements while the nurse tries to deal with them; replaying the taped segment should help both to see where communication could have been clearer and more consistent.

Role-Playing or Simulated Situations

At the end of this section, the reader will find role-playing or simulated exercises that can be used to practice assertive individual and group behaviors as supervisor or administrator, supervisee, colleague, or in situations with clients and their families. Assert (Clark, 1976) is a simulation game that can be used by groups of nurses to practice assertive behaviors.

In these exercises, as in the ones above, the nurse is given a chance to practice the assertive behavior before being placed in the anxiety-provoking environment of the work setting. Such practice can often be more easily transferred to the work setting than concepts that have been learned from reading a book or viewing a film. Therefore, in order to become more assertive, the individual must be an active participant in learning to become more assertive.

DEALING WITH ANXIETY

As with all new behaviors, changing to a more assertive stance or participating more actively as a leader is likely to produce anxiety at first. Therefore, the nurse who hopes to become more assertive can profit from a series of relaxation and desensitization exercises.

The Worst-Thing Exercise

One way to prepare for anxiety-provoking situations is to make a mental or written summary of what one expects to happen at that time. Take the situation to its ultimate conclusion by asking, "What is the worst thing that could happen?" It may take a while to really get in touch with one's fears. Many times the anxiety about the worst thing is due to a fear of being rejected, laughed at, not being liked, or being retaliated against. Once the hidden fear is out in the open, it can be examined. For example, the nurse can look at the fear and ask such questions as: "So what if everyone doesn't like me for my behavior?" "Do I really expect to be able to please everyone?" "If I do, how realistic is this?"

Devising Your Own Role-Playing

When the nurse has difficulty going through the worst-thing exercise alone, role-playing can be devised to locate the ultimate source of anxiety, as well as to practice dealing with the anxiety-provoking situation before it occurs. For example, if one's fear is speaking in front of a group, several friends can be brought together to play the group. The anxious nurse can try to speak to the group and then describe what went on inside—how he or she felt, what he or she anticipated, and so forth. Then, the nurse can switch roles with one of the group members and sit and listen while someone else speaks to the group. Switching roles can give the nurse a sense of how others might feel listening to a speaker, as well as give ideas about how to (or not to) speak to a group by the way the other member speaks.

By using this method, the nurse and the group can anticipate any snags that could occur in the actual situation. Also, by actually listening to oneself speak to a nonthreatening group, receiving feedback from the group about how one is doing, and thinking about how to speak to the real group, the nurse can begin to feel more confident. Group members might come up with suggestions the nurse never thought of, such as, "Look us straight in the eye when you talk to us" or "Try sounding more sure of yourself when you say that."

Tape recordings can be combined with role-playing if it seems important for the nurse to hear how he or she sounds. Many times nurses are not aware of how timid, angry, or guilty they sound until they hear their own voices.

Relaxation Exercises

A third skill the nurse can use to decrease anxiety before encountering an anxiety-provoking situation is relaxation. Certain exercises can help people physically relax their bodies. When anxiety occurs, body musculature becomes more rigid, pulse and respiration may increase, and there is a general tightening up. Relaxation exercises teach the body that there is nothing to become tense and threatened about. The first step is to select a pleasant, relaxing scene. The next step is to practice picturing that scene until it can be visualized mentally at will. Next, make an effort to tense up all of the muscles and then relax them, letting all the tension out of the body when exhaling. (This exercise should be done in a quiet room when no one else is present).

When the nurse can relax completely and picture the pleasant scene, he or she is ready to begin thinking about the steps that will occur in the anxiety-provoking situation. For example, if the problem is speaking to a group, the learner can imagine getting ready to leave home to speak to the group; if no anxiety is experienced yet, the learner can visualize getting into the car and driving to the place where the group will meet. The learner takes the imagined upcoming situation step by step, stopping whenever anxiety is experienced, and relaxing muscle tension, and thinking about the pleasant, calming scene. By repeating this process, the learner will eventually be able to proceed mentally through the entire upcoming event without experiencing anxiety. Such prepractice will reduce the possibility of becoming highly anxious in the actual situation, although this relaxation exercise can also be used at that time as well. Whenever the feeling of anxiety starts to seem overwhelming, the person says, "Think of the pleasant scene" while taking deep, slow breaths and letting tension out with exhalation.

ROLE-PLAYING SITUATIONS

Think of assertive responses to the following management situations:

1   You ask a nurse to help out with an assignment, saying, "We're all pitching in to help today." He or she does not answer you. You go to work with another client, and then hear a commotion in the hall. You go to see what has happened, and you find that the nurse is in the middle of the commotion. You ask what happened, and he or she begins to yell at you in front of clients and doctors.

2   You work with a clerk who "likes to do things her own way." The rule is that clients in the clinic are called on a first-come basis; some people arrive late and try to manipulate the clerk into being seen before

the others who have been waiting. You arrive on the scene just as the clerk and the clients are about to come to blows.

3 Another nurse is always asking favors of you. He or she tries to appear very busy and you feel sorry for her and so do his or her work. After you finish, you feel exploited and wish you could tell the nurse to do his or her own work since you both have equally taxing assignments.

4 You have just been placed in charge of a health clinic. The nursing aides are speaking loudly and are not concerned with the clients. They are always challenging your authority. When you ask them to do things, they refuse. You go to your immediate supervisor for assistance; he says he will back you up, but then does not follow through. You feel the supervisor should give you some support by clarifying the job description of all of the workers.

5 You are the only nurse on an interdisciplinary planning committee. You notice that the doctor always calls the committee members by their first names, but is referred to as "Doctor." She seems to have her own objectives for health care, but has not considered the fact that the other committee members may have relevant ideas to contribute.

SUMMARY

Assertiveness in nursing is setting goals, acting on those goals in a clear and consistent manner, and taking responsibility for the consequences of one's actions. Assertiveness differs from aggressiveness in that the latter means trying to control or manipulate another person; the latter may also lead to retaliative behavior.

Nurses have a difficult time being assertive because of their socialization, nursing education, and the norms of the health care system. Nurses can learn to be more assertive in their nonverbal communication, in their verbal communication, and even in their more complex interactions. The nurse can increase assertiveness by thinking through work goals, assessing assertiveness, setting goals, changing work habits, and actively practicing assertiveness.

REFERENCES

Burnside, I. M. 1971. Peer supervision: a method of teaching. *Journal of Nursing Education* 10,3:15–18.

Clark, C. C. 1976. Assert: a simulation game to teach assertiveness. (Available from the author, P.O. Box 132, Sloatsburg, N.Y. 10974.)

———. 1977. Learning outcomes in a simulation game for associate degree nursing students. *Health Education Monographs* 5 (Supplement) 1:18–27.

———. 1978. *Assertive Skills for Nurses*. Wakefield, Ma.: Contemporary.

Fagin, C. M. 1975. Nurses' rights. *American Journal of Nursing* 75,1:82–85.

Fensterheim, H.: and J. Baer, 1975. *Don't say yes when you want to say no*. New York: Dell.

Nehren, J. G.: and M. L. Larson, 1968. Supervised supervision. *Perspectives in Psychiatric Care* 6,1:25–27.

Smith, M. J. 1975. *When I say no, I feel guilty*. New York: Bantam.

Stein, L. 1968. The doctor-nurse game. *American Journal of Nursing* 68,1:101–105.

Taubman, B. 1976. *How to become an assertive woman*. New York: Simon and Schuster.

Thomstad, B. 1975. Changing the rules of the doctor-nurse game. *Nursing Outlook* 23,7:422–427.

Chapter 8

Humanizing Nursing Care

Shelley Van Kempen

OBJECTIVES

After studying this chapter, the learner will:

- List the components of dehumanization and humanization
- List those factors that currently contribute to the dehumanization of nursing care
- Define primary nursing
- Compare team or functional nursing and primary nursing in relation to:
  —organizational pattern
  —continuity of care
  —accountability
  —client and nurse satisfaction
  —degree of humanization accomplished

There can be little doubt that hospitalization is a dehumanizing experience. Both the lay and professional literature abound with examples of uncaring and inhumane treatment of those who come to our hospitals seeking help (for example, Kern 1977; Nelson 1973; Hall 1968). This chapter will explore the dehumanization and humanization of nursing care and suggest an approach that will enhance the latter.

DEHUMANIZATION VERSUS HUMANIZATION

After an extensive review of sociological and psychological literature, Leventhal (1975) has suggested six aspects of dehumanization in hospitals: (1) being viewed as a physical object or thing (depersonalization), (2) the indifference of others to one's subjective experiences, (3) doubt and confusion arising from events that are not understood, (4) loss of the ability to plan for and cope with the situation (powerlessness), (5) impaired communication due to either an inability to describe one's subjective experience or an anticipation of criticism and negative response from others, and (6) emotional distress that arises from and exacerbates all of the above factors.

One journal article was written by a physician-patient who was made to suffer much of what he himself had previously inflicted on clients (Kern 1977). His major problem was not with the physical care he received but with the inhuman attitudes of the health professionals. Dr. Kern discusses a number of dehumanizing events, including: prolonged waiting for pain medication; sleeping and eating routines that were totally alien to his usual lifestyle; taking of his vital signs in a ritualistic way that reminded him of a mechanic checking the working parts of a machine; "partial" bed baths with cold, scummy water given by someone who really was not interested in the "unreachable" parts; and noise around the clock, including the 4:30 A.M. testing of the public address system. Slate (1966, p. 122) discusses the "law of inverse communication," that is, "the unwillingness of the nurses to tell you anything except what you do not want to know."

Not surprisingly, it is usually one or more of these dehumanizing factors that is responsible for the "difficult," "problem," "uncooperative," or "unpopular" client. With tongue-in-cheek, Peterson (1967) suggests several dehumanizing tactics that are guaranteed to create "difficult" clients; for example, refer to clients not by name but by room number; let clients know that they can make no decisions regarding their care; *tell* clients how they feel and refer to them in the third person in their presence ("Don't you think he needs another blanket? He looks cold").

Many articles (Peterson 1967; Nelson 1973; Lorber 1975) list the types of clients who are likely to become the victims of dehumanizing attitudes or behavior on the part of the nursing staff and thus "problems":

those with chronic or serious illnesses; those who are unpleasant, angry, depressed, or complaining; those who are incapacitated or mentally ill; and those who are dying. Regardless of the nursing staff, simply entering a hospital is a dehumanizing experience.

Howard (1975) suggests several aspects of humanization in hospitals: recognition of individual worth, recognition of individual uniqueness, recognition of the wholeness of a person, freedom of action, equality of status, and shared decision making. These aspects seem contradictory to the position that clients find themselves in when they enter a hospital.

Recognition of Individual Worth   The individual's sense of worth and self-confidence is decreased when illness strikes. As one is relieved of social responsibilities and assumes the sick role, much of one's sense of identity is dissipated. Also, failing physical health can be a severe blow to one's self-esteem.

Recognition of Individual Uniqueness   What's in a name? Everything. Yet when clients enter the health care system, they are strangers and are rarely called or addressed by name. They are generally given a label that immediately puts them into the class of "patients:" "Dr. Smith's new patient," "The new patient in 406," or "The hernia for the OR tomorrow." Their uniqueness is lost.

In fact, even the word *patient* connotes a loss of individuality. Clients are intelligent, self-directed persons who go to their lawyer, accountant, or business associate with a problem, and the two work out a solution. The professional is accountable to the client and keeps him or her informed about progress and outcomes: they consult *with* each other. A patient simply becomes one of a large group of "patients," unknowledgeable, passive, dependent, and "sick." The patient is told when to sleep, eat, bathe, have visitors, take pills, and go to the bathroom. The word *client* connotes a more collaborative relationship and recognition of the individual as a person.

Recognition of the Wholeness of a Person   The client cannot be viewed as a whole person when there is a large hospital staff to deal with: this one takes the vital signs, this one gives medications, this one does the bath, this one does range of motion exercises, this one takes care of planning the menu, and so forth. (It is partly because each of these persons needs time to "do their own thing" that hospital routines are so rigid). No *one* person understands what the client is really like or what his or her response to illness is. If communication between all these people is a problem, and it generally is, the situation is even worse. And if it is difficult for the hospital personnel to keep each other informed, it is equally difficult for the client to keep track of what's going on.

Example
Ms. F. was to be scheduled in the OR for the removal of a scalp abscess. She was very apprehensive about it. Dr. A. told her it would be performed sometime the following week by Dr. K. Dr. K. was planning to do the procedure the next day, but had told no one about this scheduling. Resident X. came up and wrote preoperative orders for blood work, EKG, Phisohex hairwash, and shaving of the scalp. No one informed Ms. F. about any of this. That next morning two different laboratory technicians came up to draw blood. Ms. F. asked each of them what the sample was for. Both technicians said they did not know, but that the doctor had ordered it. The EKG technician replied the same way. When the nursing aide came to do the special hairwash, Ms. F. got suspicious. Her question to the aide was answered by, "I don't know. I was just told to do this." Finally, the OR technician came in to shave Ms. F.'s head. When she asked him what was going on, he told her it was for the operation the following day. Ms. F. was alarmed, began crying, and said there must be some mistake. She screamed that she wasn't ready for this operation and asked why was everyone trying to pressure her into it. The situation was eventually clarified, and the surgery was performed the following week. Meanwhile, however, Ms. F. had experienced unnecessary stress, not to mention a variety of procedures that had to be repeated the following week.

Freedom of Action   This is obviously restricted, especially in a hospital. As mentioned earlier, hospital routines leave little room for individual preferences or idiosyncrasies. Lewis (1975) calls the health care consumer a "compliant captive," an adult who has been reduced to the dependency and status of a child—and a dumb one at that. Freedom of action is related to the following two aspects.

Equality of Status and Shared Decision Making   The fact that clients and practitioners are not equals and that decision making is not usually shared is discussed in greater detail in Chapter 12. Suffice it to say that clients are powerless in our health care system; they are seldom informed about the status of their health or about the bureaucratic workings of the system. Traditionally, health care providers have been viewed as the possessors of "special" knowledge, beyond the comprehension of the average client. As a result, clients are not prepared to participate in decision making even though it is *their* lives and health that are at issue.

DEHUMANIZATION OF NURSING CARE

Nurses are as guilty as anyone else in tolerating or even promoting dehumanization. One way this is done (besides the examples already given) is through the method of delivering care to clients; at present this is typically the functional method or the team nursing method. Although we will discuss team nursing, most of its disadvantages apply to functional nursing as well because both are task-oriented rather than client-oriented. Both team and functional nursing tend to fragment the client, which is their source of dehumanization.

Functional nursing is the method that assigns nursing personnel according to tasks or functions, for example, medication, treatment, vital signs, and A.M. care. Team nursing is an effort to deliver quality nursing care by using auxiliary nursing personnel (L.P.N.s and aides) under the supervision of a registered nurse. It became popular after World War II because of the fact that there were fewer registered nurses and more auxiliary personnel (Marram et al. 1976, p. 1). Most of the nurses on the team are assigned to provide care for specific clients. However, team nursing is often combined with functional nursing on busy units so that "total patient care" or "holistic care" is not a reality in practice.

A unit organization chart under team nursing (see Figure 8-1) shows several workers who are assigned to clients and report to the team leader who, in turn, reports to the head nurse. The team leader coordinates, supervises, and evaluates the care given to clients and their response to that care.

There are three major disadvantages to this system. First, it generally deteriorates into functional nursing since the R.N. must do certain tasks (medications, treatments) that other, less skilled team members are unable to perform. Thus, less time is spent coordinating and evaluating care.

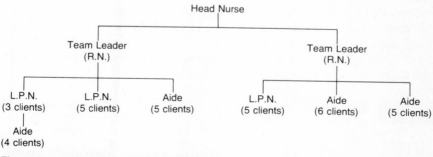

Figure 8-1 Organizational chart for team nursing.

Second, whether team or functional, there is little continuity of care. The care of the client is shared by more than one worker during each shift, which means quite a few different workers over a 24-hour period. Multiplying this by several days and taking into account days off and part-time workers, one can understand that it would be difficult for clients to keep track of just who was caring for them. This fragmentation of responsibility leads to communication barriers because clients never have enough contact with any *one* person to develop trust. It is difficult for the staff to find out what is really happening to the clients, especially when workers approach them with only one specific task in mind such as taking vital signs or giving a bath.

Lack of continuity is related to the third disadvantage—lack of accountability. Anyone who has worked as a staff nurse is acquainted with the pattern of blaming the preceding shift for the complications or inadequacies of the current shift. "If nights would only . . ." or "They should have ordered that on days!" are all-too-familiar complaints.[1] With so many different people sharing responsibility for meeting clients' needs, accountability is impossible; one can always blame someone else. This lack is especially apparent in care planning. Since no *one* person is responsible for the care plan, often it is not done; if it is done, no one utilizes it. The same thing happens with the admission assessment.

Other communications may also be a problem. Certain information is passed along when making a nursing report at the end of a shift. Besides being time-consuming, this method of communication is verbal and so it may be distorted or forgotten.[2]

Distortion may also occur in communications with other health care professionals because the message is usually transmitted through so many people. The classic example is the doctor (or social worker or physical therapist) who asks the head nurse what kind of a night the client had. There are two frequent responses: (1) The head nurse does not know because the night nurse has already left, or (2) The head nurse asks the team leader, who asks the aide, who asks the client; the reply then travels up the same hierarchy to the doctor. It is not likely that the doctor will receive accurate information, especially if several of these people have never cared for this client before. Of course, the real solution would be for the doctor to ask the client himself or herself.

---

[1] Interestingly, the night shift, as the least visible group, is usually blamed for most problems or failures.

[2] Personal experience with the change-of-shift report leads the author to conclude that the information that *is* transmitted is fragmented, incomplete, task-focused, and biased. This is the main vehicle for passing along client labels—"a pain," "obnoxious," "troublemaker," and so forth.

Team nursing does very little to promote humanization. As discussed earlier, the division of labor interferes with the process of caring for the whole person and his or her unique responses to illness, thereby decreasing the client's sense of worth. Because the client is far outnumbered by health care workers, there is no equality of status. The inability to share in the decision making and the resulting lack of freedom of action are also related to lack of accountability. These important client behaviors are restricted because, no one worker accepts responsibility for keeping the client informed (and information is required for effective decision making) and, no one person is responsible for making decisions about care (planning), and without planning there are few decisions to be shared and little freedom of action for the client.

With respect to the dehumanization of professional nursing staff, team nursing as an organizational pattern surely exacerbates what Kramer (1974) calls "reality shock." Nursing students are educated to care for the whole person, to confront all aspects of a client's response to illness. A task-oriented or fragmented approach contradicts the new graduates' self-concept. Nurses who see themselves as total-care givers will undoubtedly experience frustration and disillusionment. The components of humanization—recognition of individual worth, individual uniqueness, wholeness of the person, and so forth—are all missing for the nurse as well as the client.

PRIMARY NURSING: A HUMANIZING ALTERNATIVE

Primary nursing is a system of nursing practice where the care of a specific client is the continuous (24-hour) responsibility of one nurse from admission through discharge. The conditions that made team nursing necessary after World War II have changed; now there is an increasing number of registered professional nurses, and this has led, in part, to the development of primary nursing. But perhaps more important has been the nurses' increasing discontent with the team system.

Ciske (1974, p. 29) has listed several basic concepts in primary nursing:

1 Each client is assigned to a primary nurse, who cares for that client every day on duty for the entire length of the hospital stay.
2 The primary nurse does the assessment and plans all nursing care from admission to discharge, 24 hours a day. This information is communicated via the Kardex or other communication tools. When the primary nurse is not on duty, an associate cares for the client.

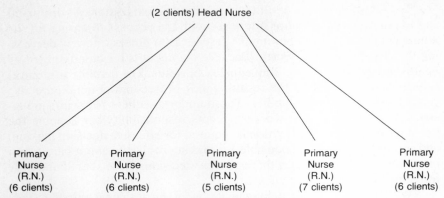

Figure 8-2 Unit organizational chart for primary nursing.

3 The client participates in his or her own care, including the identification of goals and making decisions about how to accomplish them.

One glance at a unit organizational chart under primary nursing reveals that one layer in the pyramid has been eliminated from team nursing (see Figure 8-2). Since each nurse is responsible for a select group of clients, the head nurse serves as more of a consultant, facilitator, or resource person to the primary nurses but may also carry primary clients as well.

Among the advantages of this sytem of delivering nursing care, there is substantially more continuity. The client has one person, "my nurse," who plans the client's care during the entire stay. Associate nurses on the three shifts[3] are also kept as consistent as possible. Obviously, the clients would have contact with a more manageable number of health care personnel. The clients would no longer have to begin each day by telling a new staff person all about themselves; consistency in care would enhance the clients' sense of worth.

A second advantage is that primary nursing entails having one person accountable for all aspects of a client's care. The primary nurse has the authority to plan the client's care and the responsibility to see that it is carried out. If care is not given or the results are poor, there is clearly one person—the primary nurse—who is accountable. Feedback, both *good*

---

[3]The primary nurse may be an evening or night nurse with an associate nurse during the day. However, Elpern (1977, p. 209) reports that in her experience it is difficult to carry primary clients while on the night shift because of inadequate client contact, inaccessibility of the family, and difficulty in contacting other departments or professionals about the client's care.

and *bad* is directed to the primary nurse. Primary nurses can see the direct relationship between their actions and the results; they cannot blame someone else.[4]

Communication is facilitated by primary nursing partly because of the decreased number of persons in the organizational hierarchy. Each primary nurse reports to the evening or night associate directly about the client's care. Since several staff members care for the same group of clients, it is not necessary to repeat each client's experiences over and over again. Responsibility for assessment and designing a plan of care is clearly assigned and more likely to be completed on a primary unit (Marram et al. 1976). Because the associates are responsible for following the plan of care designed by the primary nurse and the client, they are more likely to read and utilize the written care plan. Under this system, when a doctor asks what kind of a night the client had, he or she is referred directly to the client's primary nurse and the client for information. These direct lines of communication minimize the possibilities of distortion that are found in team nursing.

Primary nursing promotes the humanization of nursing care. The clients' sense of worth is increased by a feeling that they are the focus of the health care system; the expression "my nurse" indicates a certain sense of pride and security in knowing that there is one person on whom they can consistently call for help. Since primary nursing is organized around the individual person, rather than the efficient completion of tasks, clients are not viewed as pieces of a machine. The primary nurse knows the clients' reactions to all aspects of their illnesses, and so the person is viewed as a whole. As the primary nurse spends more and more time with the client and as mutual trust increases, the nurse is more aware of and able to attend to individual idiosyncrasies. There is a minimum of indifference to the client's subjective experience. Ciske (1974, p. 30) reported that with primary care, nurses are less likely to call clients "demanding" or "difficult."

When one of the stated objectives of primary nursing is carried out—to have clients participate in setting goals and making decisions—there is more freedom of action and equality of status as compared with the team method. Clients benefit from their collaboration with the primary nurse on a one-to-one basis.

It is the belief of the author that because of these humanizing factors in the primary nursing method, there is a higher level of client and staff satisfaction as compared with the team method. A comprehensive study

---

[4]It is easier to evaluate the nursing staff under the primary system since a nurse's actions and the results are more visible to the evaluator (head nurse) as well.

of both methods of nursing done by Marram et al. (1976, p. 58) found that clients perceive the primary nursing staff as performing more individualized nursing care than the team nursing staff; overall client satisfaction was significantly higher on the primary unit (Marram 1976, pp. 56–57).

Primary nurses spend much more time observing and assessing clients and their families and giving them emotional support and teaching (Marram et al. 1976, pp. 29–31). This is an important finding since traditionally health care professionals have not been held as accountable for the psychosocial care of their clients as for their physical care. This emotional support adds to the client's sense of worth.

The decreased turnover rate of nurses on primary units may indicate their higher satisfaction with this method of delivery (Spoth 1977, p. 222; Ciske 1974, p. 30). Another factor in nurses' satisfaction is their ability to practice those behaviors that they believe are most important. Two tasks that primary nurses feel are important are those that they usually complete, for example, the emotional care of families and the assessment and teaching of clients. The degree of reality shock experienced by new graduates would be less on primary units since this is the model for nursing education.

SUMMARY

The humanization of nursing care has been discussed within the framework of six factors: recognition of clients' worth, the uniqueness of the individual, viewing the client as a whole person, freedom of action, equality of status, and shared decision making. Primary nursing as a system of organizing nursing practice has been presented as an alternative to current methods that would enhance these humanizing factors.

Primary nursing is by no means a panacea. Specific problems such as development of the unit manager role, fears of overinvolvement with clients, resistance to the idea of 24-hour accountability, feelings of possessiveness about clients, and confusion about role expectations are discussed in detail by many authors (for example, Spoth 1977; Zander 1977). Despite these obstacles, primary nursing does solve some of the problems currently confronting nurses and the care they give. Table 8-1 demonstrates the positive value of primary nursing compared to team nursing with regard to humanizing factors and other variables. Implementation[5] of primary nursing is consistent with a systems point of view in that it recognizes the importance of variables that relate to the organization or environment in which care is given.

---

[5]This discussion has not dealt with *strategies* for implementation; several excellent works on this topic are listed at the end of the chapter ("Suggested Readings").

Table 8-1 Comparison of Team and Primary Nursing on Selected Variables

	Variable	Team nursing	Primary nursing
← Humanizing Factors →	Recognition of worth	Low because of task-orientation, rigid routines, fragmentation	High because of person-orientation, continuity, flexible routines
	Uniqueness of individual Wholeness of person		Increased attention to emotional needs and teaching
	Freedom of action	Limited; need to be around for team members to "do their thing" on	Increased; scheduling more individualized
	Equality of status	Client is outnumbered; has decreased status and power	One-to-one relationship with responsible nurse; has increased status and power
	Shared decision making	Lower, partly because no one person is responsible for keeping client informed	Higher; this is part of basic role conception seen as a priority one person responsible
	Communication	Complicated, indirect; possibility of distortion	Simplified, direct; less likelihood of distortion
	Care planning	Haphazard, short-term, often neglected	Over 24 hours, from admission to discharge continuous, done more often
	Responsibility	Limited to 8-hour shift	Over 24-hour period
	Accountability	Diffuse, belongs to group (team), unclear	Clear-cut, belongs to individual nurse
	Continuity	Limited due to large number and variety of care-givers	Maintained; same nurse from admission to discharge
	Nurse satisfaction	Questionable due to high turnover rates and absenteeism	*Increased; lower turnover rates Increased congruence between nursing education and service
	Client satisfaction		*Higher than with team nursing

*Findings in studies by Marram et al. (1976, p. 59).

135

REFERENCES

Armacost, Betty; Turner, Elizabeth; Martin, Mary; and Hott, Yvonne, 1974. A group of "problem" patients. *American Journal of Nursing* 74,2:289–292.

Ciske, Karen L. 1974. Primary nursing: an organization that promotes professional practice. *Journal of Nursing Administration* 4,1:28–31.

Elpern, Ellen Heid. 1977. Structural and organizational supports for primary nursing. *Nursing Clinics of North America* 12,2:205–219.

Howard, Jan. 1975. Humanization and dehumanization of health care: a conceptual view. In *Humanizing health care,* ed. Anselm Strauss and Jan Howard. New York: Wiley, pp. 57–102.

Kern, Arthur. 1977. Hospitals are no place for sick people. *Good Housekeeping* 185,111: 160–164.

Kramer, Marlene. 1974. *Reality shock.* St. Louis: Mosby.

Leventhal, Howard. 1975. The consequences of depersonalization during illness and treatment. In *Humanizing health care,* ed. by Anselm Strauss and Jan Howard. New York: Wiley, pp. 119–162.

Lewis, Edith. 1975. Health care consumer: compliant captive? *Nursing Outlook* 23,1:21.

Lorber, Judith. 1975. Good patients and problem patients: conformity and deviance in a general hospital. *Journal of Health and Social Behavior* 16,6:213–225.

Marram, Gwen; Flynn, Kathleen; Abaravich, Wendy; and Carey, Sheila. 1976. *Cost-effectiveness of primary and team nursing.* Wakefield, Mass.: Contemporary.

Nelson, Barbara Koval. 1973. The unpopular patient. *Modern Hospital* 121,2:70–72.

Peterson, Donald I. 1967. Developing the difficult patient. *American Journal of Nursing* 67,3: 522–525.

Slate, John H. 1966. De Hospitalibus Excelsior. *Atlantic* 218,7:122–123.

Spoth, Juliann. 1977. Primary nursing: the agony and the ecstasy. *Nursing Clinics of North America* 12,2:221–234.

Zander, Karen S. 1977. Primary nursing won't work . . . unless the head nurse lets it. *Journal of Nursing Administration* 7,8:19–23.

SUGGESTED READINGS

Geiger, H. Jack. 1975. The causes of dehumanization in health care and prospects for humanization. In *Humanizing Health Care,* ed. Anselm Strauss and Jan Howard. New York: Wiley, pp. 11–36.

Hall, Benita L. 1968. Human relations in the hospital setting. *Nursing Outlook* 16,3:43–45.

Hegyvary, Sue Thomas. 1977. Foundations of primary nursing. *Nursing Clinics of North America* 12,2:187–196.

Marram, Gwen D.; Schlegel, Margaret W.; and Bevis, Em O. 1974. *Primary nursing—a model for individualized care.* St. Louis: Mosby.

Romero, Mary; and Lewis, Gwendolyn. 1977. Patient and staff perceptions as a basis for change. *Nursing Clinics of North America* 12,2:205–219.

Vincent, Pauline. 1975. The sick role in patient care. *American Journal of Nursing* 75,7:1172–1173.

Chapter 9

The Clinical Specialist as Change Agent

Carolyn Chambers Clark

OBJECTIVES

After studying this chapter, the learner will:

- Define clinical specialist
- Describe ways the clinical specialist can work to effect change

DEFINITION OF A CLINICAL SPECIALIST

The Scope of Nursing Practice (1976, p. 5) defines clinical nurse specialist (CNS) as a practitioner who holds a master's degree with a concentration in specific areas of clinical nursing. The role of the CNS depends upon the needs of the client population, consumer expectations, and the clinical expertise of the specialist. The CNS must use clinical judgment to focus on the needs of the client system, and leadership skills to interface with others in the nursing and health care system. The CNS functions in a unique way applying clinical judgment and skills to client needs in order to serve as an advocate when the client is unable to cope with a particular situation or system. The CNS's basic responsibility is nursing care. Roles may change for a time, but when the CNS ceases to focus on the client for an extended period of time, the practitioner can no longer be called a CNS. "The health status of the client constitutes the reason for existence of the CNS's practice" (The Scope of Nursing Practice, 1976, p. 6). The CNS provides direct care to a select population in a specialty area of practice. Some of the roles and functions the CNS may develop to implement change are:

- Health teacher to clients
- Facilitator of the utilization of health care measures and community resources
- Regulator of external environmental factors
- Provider of educational experiences for colleagues
- Role model
- Researcher
- Consultant to colleagues and consumers
- Peer reviewer
- Collaborator with members of other disciplines
- Presenter of testimony for health care legislation
- Leader in defining problems, establishing goals, and developing ways to achieve these goals
- Improver of nursing care quality
- Coordinator of interdisciplinary services
- Member of health care delivery committees and advisory and planning groups

Which of these will be developed depends upon the CNS's assessment and intervention in system variables.

AUTHORITY AND CHANGE

One of the major reasons why the CNS is not used appropriately, which often leads to the CNS's failure to establish authority and promote change, is the assignment of the title when there is no congruence with the function(s) demanded by the work setting. The CNS may have no support system of other specialists or administrators. When the head nurse and others do not view the CNS's work as necessary or reward it, the CNS is bound to fail (Woodrow and Bell 1971, pp. 23–28). In the traditional organizational structure, the CNS may face interpersonal problems. Some nurses may feel threatened by a new breed of nurse who develops new clinical roles and functions. This threat can be decreased if the CNS can demonstrate superior knowledge of client needs and resources. However, if the system will not allow the specialist to demonstrate competence, failure will often ensue.

Walton (1973, p. 687) suggests that this factor can be mitigated by preliminary planning. A careful analysis of the work setting and its receptivity to the changes necessary for the successful entry of a CNS into the system can reduce resistance to change. This assumes a well-defined framework with a delineation of authority related to both administrative and clinical control.

The issue of administrative versus clinical control of the environment is a hotly debated issue. Alexander (1973, p. 205) argues that CNSs derive their authority from clinical competence and a knowledge of human needs, whereas administrators and managers of nursing derive their authority from a broad knowledge of the principles of planning and decision making, an understanding of nursing practice, and skills in communication. Parkis (1974b, p. 24) suggests that when the CNS is not given line authority, his or her success depends upon his or her personal relationship with the supervisor. Georgopoulos and Christman (1970, p. 1033) described an experiment in role definition in which CNSs were given formal authority and responsibility for clinical nursing practice on their respective units. They had no teaching or administrative responsibilities. They could bypass the (administrative) nursing supervisor under whom they worked by going directly to the director of nursing service whenever they chose to do so.

Parkis (1974b, p. 28) states that a CNS who has no formal authority over the direction of client care is an administrative waste of time and money. She also says that there is still confusion in defining the role, determining the level of function, and placing the clinical specialist in nursing systems.

Shea (1975) suggests that the CNS replace the nursing supervisor. Lysaught (1974, p. 336) supports this view; he summarizes why the traditional nursing supervisor role is dysfunctional:

1　He or she is drawn away from direct care (leading to loss of clinical expertise).
2　He or she has little influence over subordinates because they have no authority to reward or punish (decisions are made at a higher level).
3　There is incongruence between the concerns of the personnel and systems maintenance and the concerns of the staff and clients.
4　There is discontinuity between the hospital goals and the client care goals.

One solution to this problem is to discard the role of the (administrative) supervisor and allow the head nurse to assume some of his or her functions and prerogatives. This does not solve the problem of clinical supervision, however, since the head nurse does not have advanced preparation in a clinical speciality.

Barrett (1972, p. 524) reports the use of a clinical specialist in this manner. The head nurse position was eliminated and replaced by a CNS with administrative responsibility for the nursing care of small groups of clients. In this study the CNS had 24-hour responsibility for fifteen to eighteen clients, provided direction and supervision of nursing personnel, gave direct care in terms of assessing needs and formulating care plans, and established a collegial relationship with the medical staff. Although Barrett writes that the CNS functioned with a great deal of autonomy, it was within a system where the CNS reported to both a department supervisor and the director of nursing.

Shea (1975, pp. 10–11) states that one principle of good management is to have the fewest levels of management and to have a short chain of command. An ideal management situation is one where the client has access to the director of nursing through the R.N. and CNS. By contrast, in rigid, hierarchically structured hospitals, the following levels must be addressed: client to aide or L.P.N., to R.N., to team leader, to head nurse, to supervisor, to assistant director of nursing, to director of nursing, to associate executive director, to executive director, to president, to chairman of the board. Shea (1975, p. 15) also points out that in order for the ideal system to work, the CNS must be given responsibility and authority for care, while a service unit management team has the responsibility and authority for non-nursing duties.

Knowledgeable directors of nursing may not question the specialist's competence in clinical judgment or practice. They may, however, question the CNS's management or leadership skills. Shea (1975, p. 16) counters that the CNS has had extensive education and experience in interpersonal relationships which is at the very heart of nursing and management. Gilbert's research (1975, p. 125) supports the view that graduate students in nursing have a high potential for leadership and management.

ACCOUNTABILITY AND CHANGE

The major difficulty in working out the accountability issue is the fact that the CNS role was not designed to fit into the bureaucratic, hierarchical system that is usually found in health care institutions (Stevens 1977, p. 77). Stevens clarifies this issue by discussing professional and administrative authority and the relationship of authority to accountability. Professional authority is power or influence achieved through a response of peers; administrative authority is granted to a position rather than to a particular individual. "Professional authority applies to every competent clinical specialist, while administrative authority depends upon her job description and place in the organization" (Stevens 1977, p. 77).

When the CNS has only professional authority, the director of nursing should hold him or her accountable only for direct care, since the staff use of the specialist's expertise depends upon interpersonal variables. For the CNS who functions under this system of authority, change is related to the outcome of client care. An improved outcome is expected; the CNS must be able to establish the fact that care improved as a result of his or her intervention and that it was efficient (or beneficial in terms of cost). For example, to have a CNS give a bed bath may result in improved care, but the crucial point is whether it is efficient with respect to using the CNS's time.

Stevens (1977, p. 78) stresses that it is illogical for a director of nursing to hire a CNS at a professional authority level (staff position) and expect him or her to function as both an interpersonal specialist and client care specialist. This is illogical because teaching complex interpersonal skills is seldom part of the CNS's education, except in some psychiatric-mental health graduate programs; the potential probably remains undeveloped in nonpsychiatric programs.

On the other hand, if the director of nursing hires a CNS at an administrative authority level (line position), the CNS is expected to have the same accountability as a line manager; this requires additional management skills which many CNS educational programs do not offer. Management and clinical tasks will then vie for the specialist's time. "A clinical specialist cannot carry the same administrative tasks as other managers and still have a special impact on bedside care; this discounts the reality of administrative demands (Stevens 1977, p. 78).

It is this seemingly unresolvable issue that places both the CNS and the nursing director in a dilemma. If the CNS is placed in a staff position he or she is (at least) somewhat subject to line management decisions. If the CNS is placed in a line position, he or she has less time for client care. The dilemma for the director of nursing is that he or she wants to have the CNS function totally independently (despite the illogicality of individual independence in a bureaucratic system) and to hold the CNS accountable for his or her actions. Stevens (1977, pp. 78–79) suggests several ways to deal with these dilemmas, thus allowing the CNS to function more effectively as a change agent:

1   The CNS should make a complete assessment of his or her own expectations for work, the congruence between his or her clinical skills and the work environment, and his or her interpersonal skills before accepting a staff position.

2   The director of nursing should assess his or her own expectations for the CNS, the work, and the interpersonal variables to make sure that the CNS is not being hired for an impossible task.

3   The director of nursing should be aware that it may be impossible to assess the congruence between the CNS's interpersonal skills and the needs and relationship skills of the other staff members, and should realize that hiring a CNS at a staff level with coordinator and consultative responsibilities is a risk.

4   Before accepting a position, the CNS should demand an opportunity to sit down with the director of nursing to identify mutually acceptable areas of accountability.

5   Before hiring a CNS, the director of nursing should agree to sit down with the CNS to work out areas of accountability.

FEEDBACK AS CHANGE

Nadler (1976, pp. 177–186) discusses ways in which change can be effected through survey feedback, and this applies to the change agent role of the CNS. The idea of using feedback to bring about change is based on systems theory; adaptive systems are self-correcting—they make use of data about their outputs to correct system functions. Feedback can affect behavior by providing information about performance that implies what corrections should be made and that there is a need to search for new behaviors; it also provides information about goal setting and goal attainment.

If the CNS can inform a group or organization about its output (feelings, perceptions, client care), cues about problems in its human system can be delineated, new ways to deal with these problems can be sought, and motivation for improvement can be generated. In order to use survey feedback effectively, the CNS ought to consider Nadler's suggestions:

1   The group or organization should participate in collecting data. Usually, a questionnaire is developed and administered to appropriate individuals.

2   Diagnosis, feedback, and action should focus on the ongoing work group.

3   Feedback should start at the top of the organization and work down through subsystems.

4   The group or subsystem should participate in the process of analyzing feedback as a way to reduce resistance and reinforce action.

5   The group should be convened to discuss the results of the survey feedback and how it can secure help for its operation.

6   The questionnaire or survey should be readministered as an evaluative tool and as a basis for continued intervention.

The CNS as a feedback consultant can affect the resistance or acceptance of data. It has been shown that meetings are more effective in producing acceptance than are written reports. Having the CNS in a line
position (with administrative authority) may lead to more satisfied personnel since the work group may perceive that "this is important business." If the CNS does not have administrative authority, he or she can
arrange to have a nurse who is in a line position attend the meeting. Acceptance of feedback and satisfaction with the process are more likely to
occur in members who attend more than one meeting. It is wise for the
CNS to assess relevant system issues before the feedback sessions since
the members are more likely to reveal information that may be threatening
when the consultant perceives relevant data (Alderfer and Brown 1972,
pp. 456–460). Even if the CNS is in an administrative authority position,
it may be helpful to work with an outside consultant or a CNS from a
different work area; mixed teams of outside and inside consultants seem
to be the most effective in helping the feedback process. Also, the CNS
may choose to lead an initial peer group meeting, followed by an interdisciplinary group meeting, since interpersonal issues may come up more
easily and problems are often solved in this two-step process (Alderfer
and Holbrook 1973, pp. 437–464). If the CNS plans to use feedback as a
tool for change, he or she should remember that organizations are
dynamic systems that exist over time and have regular cycles of events;
feedback should be integrated with the regular cycles of the operating
system.

ERRORS COMMONLY MADE BY CHANGE AGENTS

In initiating change, the novice as well as the seasoned change agent is apt
to make mistakes. Reddin, an organization change agent, shares the following list of his own errors: initiating change from the bottom up, creating a change overload, raising expectations beyond what is possible, allowing inappropriate attachment, becoming trapped in one part of the
organization, changing only a subsystem, using behavioral instead of structural interventions, losing professional detachment, assuming that a
change is needed, and failing to seek help (1977, pp. 33–41). Some (and
possibly all) of these errors will be exemplified in the following section
"Clinical Specialists at Work."

When the CNS is approached by a staff person who is speaking for
another person (often his or her supervisor), the specialist can make a
change process error by trying to effect a bottom-to-top change. Instead,
the CNS ought to insist on talking to and working with the other person
and not accept the excuse that that person is too busy, does not need help,
or can work out the problem alone. The CNS who attempts to initiate too

many changes at one time or who tries to make even a small change in a rigid system may be making the change process mistake of change overload. Ongoing discussions with members of a system or subsystem can unfreeze rigid systems and decrease the potential for overload and resistance.

One of the easiest mistakes to make is to raise expectations beyond what is possible. The novice CNS is often enthusiastic and idealistic about what can be accomplished in a short period of time. However planned and agreed-upon progressive step changes over a three-to-four year period can reduce the possibility of this mistake. Short-term system change frameworks are often destined for failure since such expectations may not be in line with what is possible.

The CNS's relationship with the client or system is an important element in the success or failure of an intervention. When the CNS takes the role of a witty companion or pal, the client may be confused by any behaviors that are inconsistent with these role behaviors. Any attempts made by the CNS to initiate change may then be met with incredulity or increased resistance. The CNS should, therefore, have a consistent relationship and act as a change agent.

Multiple entry into a system is part of an effective change strategy. The CNS who sides with the nursing staff against the nursing or medical administration will be viewed as an isolate, scapegoat, or traitor at a later time when events require improved relationships with the administration. Developing relationships at many levels within the system decreases the possibility of becoming trapped in or by one part of the organization. Subsystem personnel may give the CNS clues about where other entry levels might be made by identifying whom the client is angry with (Reddin, 1977, p. 37).

If the CNS works out a new system with the nursing staff, but neglects to communicate important information about the procedure to other disciplines or clients, change is often knowingly (or unknowingly) resisted. Reddin (1977, p. 37) suggests that specific measurable objectives should be identified and agreed to by both the subsystem and adjacent subsystems so that change will not impair other relationships in other subsystems.

Incorrectly assessing the source of a problem can result in an inappropriate change intervention. If the CNS identifies a conflict between subsystems, the source may be at the individual, role, or skill level. Confusing behavioral difficulties with a problem in structure or skills can result in an error. For example, if the CNS decides that the source of a conflict is unclear goals and intervenes to clarify them when actually the source is poor communication skills, there will be an ineffective change.

If the CNS intervenes because of his or her own feelings of depression, anger, confusion, or anxiety, or the need to be liked, praised, or unusually successful, professional detachment is sacrified. Each CNS should be aware of danger signals indicating impediments to the change process.

Another common mistake is to assume that change in and of itself is better than no change. It is important to assess the need for change; Reddin states that new is not necessarily better than old. He says that initiating change merely for its own sake can be a change agent error (1977, p. 39).

People in the helping professions are seldom likely to seek help themselves. Perhaps this is because they try to meet their own dependency needs or need to be cared for by caring for others. Helpers in the psychiatric-mental health area have often been advised to seek clinical supervision upon graduation. If they do so, they are more likely to be able to deal with difficulties and to recognize failure. The CNS may be in a particularly difficult position because he or she is assumed to be an expert, and others may convey the expectation that an expert ought not to need assistance or help. In fact, the CNS may need help from peers in order to maintain an accurate perception of the system and change difficulties. Although peers, too, may distort or omit important data, they often do so in different areas than the CNS might, and so their inputs can add a useful perspective.

CLINICAL SPECIALISTS AT WORK

Individual clinical specialists work differently depending upon their skills, system variables, and their ability to coordinate the two. When the CNS can assess the system correctly, enter it with power and authority, and provide needed resources, constructive change usually occurs.

Huether et al. (1973) report the work of a team of clinical specialists in the University of Utah Hospital Nursing Service Department. They stressed the importance of collaboration with one another. The CNSs felt free to ask each other for assistance in caring for a client or solving a problem. They held clinical rounds twice a month to share care information and to learn how to collaborate together. They invited head nurses to attend their meetings if clients on their units were being discussed. Through these discussions, they learned that it was essential to give clinical and emotional support to the head nurses on all units. One suggestion that came out of these meetings was that the CNSs develop a way of offering their services to nursing units and especially those that had no specialist assigned to them.

The CNSs reviewed the needs for clinical services within all nursing units and reevaluated the daily activities and demands of the group. Through this process, they decided to offer two CNSs to each unit, one who would provide primarily psychiatric-mental health assistance and the other who would assist with physiologic problems. The assignment of pairs was based on the nature of the nursing care problems and the expertise of the specialists. Each pair arranged with the unit staff to meet together weekly or upon request.

Initially all CNS teams had to spend a great deal of time clarifying their roles. Among other things, they made sure that the head nurses and assistant directors of nursing were responsible for the unit budget, staffing, and coordination of support services; and they demonstrated they could use their advanced knowledge and skill to help the unit staff. The CNSs identified the following five phases in the acceptance and utilization of team services:

1 A mutual agreement by the head nurse and nursing staff that a clinical specialist team would work together to improve nursing care.
2 Identification of the mutual behavioral expectations of the staff and clinical specialist teams.
3 An initial collaboration and testing of the mutual and divergent goals of the staff and team members.
4 An evaluation of the team services.
5 A mutual understanding and acceptance of the team services.

The CNS at the University of Utah identified four ways to assist staff: consultation, teaching, referral, and direct care. At first, the staff requested teaching by the teams; this was interpreted but not verbalized by the CNS as safe and comfortable because the student-teacher role was known to all participants. In time, as an understanding of the team function developed, the nurses learned how to use the consultation process; from this process emerged teaching, direct care, and referral.

The CNS teams provided learning experiences for the staff by helping them identify their learning needs, select appropriate learning methods, and evaluate their learning experiences. All experiences were individualized, thereby making inservice education decentralized. Often, staff members observed a CNS performing a complex nursing skill such as using the stethoscope to evaluate breath sounds postoperatively. The staff then requested assistance in learning how to use the stethoscope in this manner.

When there was a complex or difficult care problem, the CNS and the staff decided whether the specialist should provide the care. If the decision was yes, the specialist worked in this capacity either alone or with a staff member at the bedside. When the CNS provided the care, he or she was responsible on a 24-hour basis and was obliged to communicate with the staff. This mode of interaction allowed the University of Utah specialists to model appropriate practice by means of discussion and demonstration. It was also possible for the specialist to demonstrate the value of applying appropriate knowledge to improve the client's health. It was believed that the specialist was necessary in situations where there were multiple and complex variables and where a comprehensive care plan needed to be developed. Indirectly, the CNS conveyed the importance of continued learning and evaluation in nursing practice. The specialist team provided needed information about available community facilities or services that would be important for discharge planning. They also assisted the staff in considering and using hospital services that had been overlooked.

These teams seemed to be successful in part because the director of nursing defined, defended, and supported their roles. Also, the head nurses helped to plan how to meet care needs and accepted (at least intellectually) the concept of working with a CNS.

The experience of the CNSs at the University of Utah Hospital is quite different from the author's clinical specialist experience as a graduate student (Chambers 1967) in an inpatient service that was part of a community mental health center (Clark 1968, 1972, 1975, 1976), in a general hospital (Clark 1973), and in two community health nursing services (Clark 1978). None of these experiences met the ideal conditions described by Huether et al. (1973). In her first experience, the author functioned as an intern with no administrative support or authority. Any change that may have occurred in the system during that time was probably due to the interpersonal relationship between the CNS trainee and the head nurse.

In the author's next experience as a CNS, she was hired to work as a specialist, although the director of nursing did not have a line for that position. Within six months, the director of nursing was exerting strong pressure for the author to serve in the role of staff nurse. In this situation, the major problems seemed to be the lack of agreement as to what was expected of the CNS, a lack of administrative support for the CNSs activities, and a lack of staff preparation for work with a specialist.

In her third CNS experience (Clark 1968, 1972, 1975, 1976), the author was hired to work as a specialist, and there was verbal (if not actual) support of the role. Again, the staff was not prepared to accept the idea of working with a CNS. The author carved out a role based on her interpersonal relationships with the head nurse and other staff members and on her ability to provide support and learning experiences for the nursing staff. A major difficulty on this job was the lack of peer support. When other CNSs were hired, the author participated in monthly collaboration meetings with these other specialists. Another problem was to correct the misconceptions held by members of other disciplines regarding the CNSs ability to be a primary therapist with individuals, groups, and families (Clark 1968). Additional assessments and planned interventions had to be developed to deal with the cognitive and interpersonal styles of a client population that was not white or middle class. Another adaptation demanded by this particular community health nursing service was the need for short-term treatment rather than a long-term, one-to-one relationship that had been emphasized in the author's graduate education.

Out of necessity, a method was developed for working with large, short-term groups of highly disturbed clients. On the author's first day as a CNS, a client hanged himself in the bathroom. The CNS gathered the unit clients together to discuss the incident. Subsequently, an ongoing group was begun to deal with emergency and daily problems of hospital life. Before the group, unit procedure called for a psychiatrist, psychologist, or social worker to interview a client. The group seemed to meet a need, lessen anxiety, and change the atmosphere of the unit. The group was led five times a week by the author and a clinical psychologist, but as more unit activities became available, the group only met three times a week.

Starting such a group led to certain staff and client resistance, which typically follows the introduction of change in a social system. It took more than a year for the group to be accepted as a viable treatment modality, evaluation tool, or method of socialization. At appointed group times, psychiatric residents often scheduled sessions with their clients, and the staff members acted as if the group did not exist. The coleaders volunteered information during staff conferences and added notes on the nursing Kardex. Within a year, the ward chief began to ask about the behavior of individual group members and staff conferences were used to discuss a client's behavior in the group as part of the predischarge evaluation (Clark 1972; Clark 1976a). Because there was a rapid turnover of both staff and clients (with many readmissions), the unit often had an atmosphere of apathy and hopelessness. Consequently, the author began to make suggestions for counteracting these feelings (Clark 1975).

Although many system difficulties could be worked through in an individual manner, many could not or were not dealt with appropriately. One difficulty was in off-unit consultations. There was no nursing administration support for CNS visits to other units. There was no discussion about the structure of the visits or what would be accomplished. Staff members on the other units were not informed about the CNSs consultation function, and they did not know how to work with a consultant. Although the nursing administrators seemed to approve of consultation from an intellectual point of view, they obviously had mixed feelings about it since the author had difficulty meeting with them to plan a consultation format. These mixed feelings were undoubtedly communicated to the nurses working on the units. It appeared that the nursing supervisor decided that her staff needed mental health consultation with regard to a particular client, and so she called the assistant director of psychiatric nursing, who conveyed the message to the psychiatric mental health nursing specialist. This indirect chain of command was indicative of the type of management within this system. Requests for assistance were erratic and often of an emergency nature; this type of request obviously could not be met within a structured consultation format. Often, the pertinent staff members were not available on the unit when the CNS arrived, or they disparaged any consultative assistance. Possibly the behavior of the unit staff members reflected a system rift that had existed for years between medical-surgical nursing and psychiatric mental health nursing. Because the author did not take into account the larger system and its requirements for effecting change, her role as a consultant was never fully developed (Clark 1976b).

The teaching and supportive functions of the CNS were ongoing and demanding. With the continual turnover of head nurses and psychiatric residents, and the long-term employment of the aides, there was both anxiety and apathy. The author began a weekly nursing care conference. Ostensibly the purpose was to share nursing interventions, but the real strength of the group was that it provided support in an everchanging environment.

As a CNS, the author has also been a communication consultant (Clark 1973) to nurses on various units of a general hospital and to community health nurses in two agencies (Clark 1978). This work led to the development of a consultation presentation guide and a form for the use of consultees in evaluating consultation. This work also clarified the types of problems nurses bring for mental health consultation: clients who are overly dependent, complain, refuse to comply, or belittle the nurse. Dependency, anger, and noncompliance prevail in nurse-client relationships and are reflected in consultee-consultant sessions. Much of the consultation has taken place in group settings, and this format is advantageous in that it allows nurses to observe themselves and others and to provide peer support. During the early phases of consultation the CNS must be highly verbal, have many suggestions and ideas, and be able to distinguish between solvable and unsolvable problems (Clark 1976b; Larsen and Norris 1977, p. 27).

The author's CNS role at the community health nursing services developed somewhat according to the process described by Huether (1973, pp. 691–701). At first, the community health nurses requested clinical teaching. Later, they presented case studies and asked the CNS to make evaluation home visits with them. Much later, they began to refer clients to the CNS for mental health counseling and evaluation. Throughout her work with the community health nurses, the author continued as a consultant on how to deal with clients (Clark 1978).

SUMMARY

The clinical specialist holds a master's degree with a concentration in specific areas of clinical nursing. The primary purpose of the CNS is to care for the client. It is still not clear how much clinical and administrative authority the CNS should have. Various authors suggest that the CNS should take the place (but not the role) of the head nurse or administrative supervisor. Accountability, feedback, and common change agent errors were discussed from the viewpoint of how they might be resolved. The work of several CNSs was presented.

REFERENCES

Alderfer, C. P.; and Brown, L. D. 1972. Questionnaire design in organizational research. *Journal of Applied Psychology* 56:456–460.
——; and Holbrook, J. A. 1973. A new design for survey feedback. *Education and Urban Society* 5:437–464.
Alexander, Edythe L. 1973. Foreword: symposium on management and supervision of patient care. *Nursing Clinics of North America* 8,2:203–208.
Barrett, Jean. 1972. The nurse specialist practitioner: a study. *Nursing Outlook* 20,8:525–527.
Bell, Judith A.; and Woodrow, Mary. 1971. Clinical specialization: conflict between reality and theory. *Journal of Nursing Administration* 2,5(November–December): 23–28.
Burd, Shirley F. 1966. The clinical specialization trend in psychiatric nursing. Ed.D. dissertation, Rutgers University.
——. 1973. Clinical practice issues in mental health nursing. In *Contemporary issues in mental health nursing,* ed. Madeleine Leininger. Boston: Little, Brown, pp. 111–124.
Cahoon, M. C. 1977. Developing clinical specialist roles. *Nursing Mirror* 144:66–68.
Chambers, Carolyn. 1967. Nurse leadership during crisis situations on a psychiatric ward. *Perspectives in Psychiatric Care* 5,1:29–35.
Clark, Carolyn Chambers. 1968. Creating a role as clinical specialist in community mental health; an experiential view. Paper presented to Rutgers University Symposium on the role of the clinical specialist in community mental health, November 2, 1968, at Rutgers University, New Brunswick, New Jersey.
——. 1972. A social systems approach to short-term psychiatric care. *Perspectives in Psychiatric Care* 10,4:178–183.
——. 1973. The clinical specialist as communication consultant. *Supervisor Nurse* 4,4:20–27.

————. 1975. Tactics for counteracting staff apathy and hopelessness on a psychiatric ward. *Journal of Psychiatric Nursing* 133:3–5.

————. 1976a. The process of establishing inpatient, short-term groups. *Group Process* 6:129–139.

————. 1976b. Psychiatric-mental health consultation with nurses. Paper presented to the New York State Nurses Association Convention. October 11–15, 1976, Liberty, New York.

————. 1978. *Mental health aspects of community health nursing.* New York: McGraw-Hill.

Clark, E. Louise. 1977. A model of nurse staffing. *Journal of Nursing Administration* 7,2:22–27.

Cleland, Virginia. 1972. Nurse clinicians and nurse specialists: an overview. In *Three challenges to the nursing profession: selected papers from the 1972 ANA convention.* New York: American Nurses Association.

DeMeyer, Joanna. 1972. A nurse consultant in action. *Journal of Nursing Administration* 2,3:42–45.

Duberley, J. 1976. The clinical nurse specialist. *Nursing Times* 72:1794–1795.

Georgopoulos, Basil S.; and Christman, Luther. 1970. The clinical nurse specialist: a role model. *American Journal of Nursing* 70,5:1030–1039.

Gilbert, Marie. 1975. Personality profiles and leadership potential of medical-surgical and psychiatric nursing graduate students. *Nursing Research* 24:125–130.

Huether, Sue E.; Powell, Anne Hahn; Vaughan, Beth Ann; Evans, Dale F.; and Cole, Sandra Wistrom. 1973. Team services of a clinical specialist group. *Nursing Clinics of North America* 8,4:691–701.

Larsen, Judith K.; and Norris, Eleanor L. 1977. Consultation to mental health agencies: what makes it work or not? *Innovations* 4,2:25–28.

Lysaught, Jerome. 1974. *Action in nursing.* New York: McGraw-Hill.

Marcus, J. 1976. Nursing consultation: a clinical specialty. *Journal of Psychiatric Nursing* 14:29–31.

Mott, Basil J. 1976. Who should manage health services: implications of decentralization. *American Journal of Public Health* 66,12:1143–1145.

Nadler, David A. 1976. The use of feedback for organizational change: promises and pitfalls. *Group and Organization Studies* 1,2:177–186.

Parkis, Ellen W. 1974a. The management role of the clinical specialist. Part 1. *Supervisor Nurse* 5,9(September):45–51.

————. 1974b. The management role of the clinical specialist. Part 2. *Supervisor Nurse* 5,10 (October):24–35.

Pask, E. G. 1977. Specialization in nursing. *Canadian Nurse* 73:34–35.

Reddin, W. J. 1977. Confessions of an organizational change agent. *Group and Organization Studies* 2,1:33–41.

Rotkovitch, Rachel, ed. 1976. *Quality patient care and the role of the clinical nurse specialist.* New York: Wiley.

The scope of nursing practice: description of practice nurse practitioner/clinician clinical nurse specialist. 1976. Mimeographed document. Kansas City, Missouri: American Nurses' Association.

Shea, Carole A. 1975. Supervision in nursing: a job for the clinical specialist. Unpublished paper. New Brunswick, N.J.: Rutgers, The State University.

Smoyak, Shirley. 1976. Specialization in nursing: from then to now. *Nursing Outlook* 24:676–681.

Stevens, Barbara J. 1977. Accountability of the clinical specialist: an administrator's view. *Nursing Digest* 5:77–79.

Walton, Minnie H. 1973. Professionals: cost and quality. *Nursing Clinics of North America* 8,4:685–689.

Woodrow, Mary; and Bell, Judith A. 1971. Clinical specialization: conflict between reality and theory. *Journal of Nursing Administration* 2,6:23–28.

Chapter 10

The Head Nurse as Manager

Carole A. Shea

OBJECTIVES

After studying this chapter, the learner will:

- Identify the position of head nurse in the organizational structure
- Describe the dual role of the head nurse
- Identify the decision-making styles used by nurse-managers
- Discuss the head nurse's relations with other members of the health care system
- List several ways to improve communication skills

LEVELS OF NURSING MANAGEMENT

Management in nursing is reflected in the organization hierarchy. At the highest level, there is a director of nursing services (sometimes called the executive director or vice president, depending upon the formal structure) who reports to the chief administrator of the organization. As head of the largest division (with the largest number of employees, accounting for 40 percent of the total budget), the nursing executive should have a title, authority, and influence appropriate for top-level management.

At the middle level of management there are nursing supervisors or department heads who report directly to the director of nursing. Supervisors are responsible for several head nurses. This satisfies the principle of span of control which limits the number of persons who can be managed effectively by one person. In some small institutions such as rural hospitals, nursing homes, or community health agencies, there is no need for middle management; head nurses are directly responsible to the top nursing executive.

At the lowest level, called *first-line management,* there is a head nurse who is responsible for the staff nurses—R.N.s., L.P.N.s, nursing aides—and the clerical staff on the unit. On units that use a team nursing assignment system, the team leader does not have an official management position but may function as a nurse-manager trainee.

In very large bureaucratic organizations, there are more levels of management since each manager takes on assistants such as associate director, assistant director, or assistant head nurse. Conversely, in small organizations there may be only one or two levels of management or possibly three levels with a few individuals at each level. Levels of management are significant for nurses because the formal structure of the organization affects nursing functions, promotion practices, career opportunities, communication patterns, professional relationships, and ultimately, personal and job satisfaction.

BECOMING A NURSE-MANAGER

All nurses are managers in the broad sense because the practice of professional nursing directly parallels the practice of management. Both practices hope to accomplish their desired results successfully and effectively (Ganong and Ganong 1976, pp. 4–5). However, nurses first become managers in the organizational sense when they occupy a position on the first-line management level. In hospitals and other large health agencies this position is that of the head nurse. Usually a nurse attains this position by promotion from within the ranks, that is, from within the group of nurses on the unit. Ideally, this promotion recognizes excellence in *both* clinical skills and leadership abilities. More often, however, the promotion is based on clinical performance alone. This frequently leads to a situation where the most competent clinical practitioners are removed from bedside care to a position at a higher organizational level where they function less effectively. Nurses have accepted their promotion in order to ad-

vance their careers and make more money, despite their personal preference to continue giving direct care. This "advancement" *away* from direct care as a means for rewarding excellence in care-giving is no longer
necessary because new roles and assignment methods, such as clinical
specialist and primary care, are being implemented to enhance clinical
career goals. Nurses now have the option of pursuing a clinical or an
administrative career with the expectation of equal status and monetary
rewards. Promotion to the position of head nurse on the basis of seniority
or years of experience is totally inadequate to the needs of today's complex health organizations.

Nurses are rarely hired from outside the organization to fill head
nurse positions because management wants head nurses to have a first-
hand knowledge of the organization system and its environment. Also,
because the head nurse position is the first step on the management lad-
der, managers use this position to reward and motivate employees. They
want to develop and evaluate talent from within the organization, with
an eye to the future growth potential of the individual and the whole system.

Promotion to first-line management from within the ranks is practiced
by both business and service organizations. However, unlike most newly
promoted business managers, who undergo a training program, or are assigned to work closely with a seasoned senior manager, the recently promoted head nurse usually has no inservice training program and no experienced colleague to work with closely after a brief orientation period.
In addition to managerial inexperience, the new head nurse probably does
not have any formal education in management theory and practice.
Nevertheless, he or she is expected to function quite competently alone
on the unit. This expectation is at variance with business practice, which
assumes that the new manager has some academic understanding but will
have an extended traineeship with a gradual increase in authority and responsibility as skills are developed and practiced in the company of others
at the same level.

Another difference between business and service organizations is in
the nature of the work at the first-line level. Business managers perform
such functions as planning, organizing, directing, coordinating, and controlling in varying degrees according to their perceived capabilities and
job descriptions. The head nurse as a manager has the unique function of
being the critical person who must turn executive plans and objectives
into concrete actions to accomplish the system's goal of delivering quality
health care. In many ways, this is the most difficult task in the organization because it is often easier to think of new ideas and solutions than to
put them into practice, given the constraints of reality. Implementing
health care directives often requires a great deal of creativity in a work

setting that expects conformity to established procedures (Plachy 1976, p. 39). Stevens (1976, p. 99) describes the head nurse as being "in the pivotal position linking nursing management to nursing care." This position is not without power. By virtue of the importance of the work in achieving organization goals and the centrality of the position (which interfaces with all the other subsystems and gives access to and control of most communication), the head nurse is a key person with power and influence. First-line business managers do not have this importance since their organizations do not depend as much on the managers' performance to achieve their objectives.

The discrepancy between the head nurse's education and his or her experience as a manager, the high expectations of the organization, and the actual importance and power of the position may produce stress and conflict unless the new head nurse is exceptionally gifted and open to learning a new role.

ROLE

To be successful and effective in this complex role, a head nurse needs a strong foundation of clinical knowledge and skills on which to base judgments and make decisions; of organizing abilities in order to perform management tasks and operations; and of interpersonal skills in order to facilitate communication and the work of others. Plachy (1976, p. 41) suggests that nurse-managers need the following qualities: technical knowledge, an action-orientation, a manner that commands respect, flexibility, an openness to the environment, inquisitiveness, and a certainty about one's place and position.

Head nurses need to have exceptional qualifications because of the difficulty in playing a dual role. The head nurse has both clinical and administrative responsibilities for which he or she must answer to two authorities—the medical staff and the nursing administration, which represents the organization. Frequently there are contradictions between professional and lay values and requirements, even when all subsystems agree on the overall goal of quality care for clients. The concept of equifinality describes a situation where final results can be achieved from different starting points and using different methods. However, strong value systems and personalities may preclude smooth management procedures. The management triad of administrator, doctor, and nurse may play out a pattern of shifting coalitions as each struggles to maintain power and define the course of action (Sills 1976, pp. 1432–1434). Figure 10-1 depicts the head nurse (in the shaded area) functioning in three spheres or systems—administrative, nursing, and medical. The management triad is superimposed to indicate coalitions. In this diagram, the head nurse is

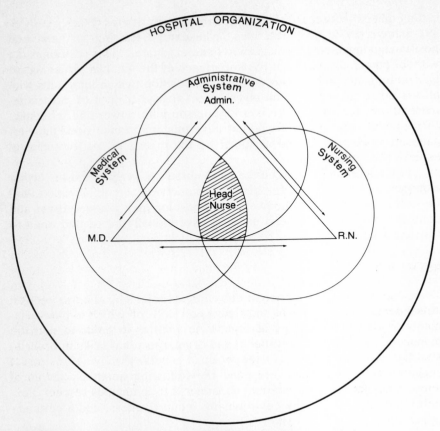

Figure 10-1 The head nurse at the center of the management triad.

located in the middle of the triad where all three systems overlap, indicating both the advantages and the disadvantages of his or her central position.

   Role conflict, which occurs when the head nurse is required to conform simultaneously to different expectations, can be resolved in constructive or destructive ways. Constructively, the head nurse can: get a written job description; clarify lines of authority; confront discrepant communications; give priority to activities that are congruent with professional values; and behave in a consistent, rational manner with all sides of the triad. Destructive activities are those that perpetuate confusion and chaos; manipulate one side against the other; and demonstrate inconsistent and immature behavior such as gossiping, scapegoating, pouting, calling in "sick," refusing to take a stand or to stick by one's own position.

The head nurse could also experience conflict if he or she does not internalize the new role as manager. For many nurses, being decisive and assertive, taking and exerting control, giving care indirectly through the work of others, and having the power to reward and sanction do not come "naturally" or are considered unfeminine. Those personality traits that help to make an excellent clinician are not necessarily useful to the successful nurse-manager. Nurses who come to the profession to do bedside nursing may have great difficulty making the transition to working with clients through others. If the head nurse was promoted because of clinical expertise, he or she might continue to perceive himself or herself primarily as a clinician and only secondarily as a manager, thereby downplaying that aspect of the role (Galloway 1974, pp. 92, 94; Stevens 1975, pp. 100–101). Nurses need time to develop a self-concept that emphasizes the strengths of the dual role of nurse and manager. Head nurses can and should give direct care to clients; this enables them to keep up their clinical skills and to keep in touch with the actual on-the-line work of the nursing practice. However, when the head nurse does give care, it should be on a planned basis and not as a stopgap measure when the staff is in short supply. If the head nurse is always filling in, this behavior undermines the manager role. The head nurse needs to be personally comfortable with the amount and kinds of direct care he or she gives, to have the respect of the nursing and medical staffs for his or her clinical abilities, and to recognize that good management contributes as much as direct care to the client's health (Stevens 1975). Internalization of the role of nurse-manager is a matter of perspective, personality, and practice.

PERFORMANCE

Ganong and Ganong (1975, pp. 16–18) have listed a variety of factors that affect the development and performance of a head nurse in a health care institution:

1 The institution's formal plan of organization.
2 The degree of responsibility and delegated authority.
3 The philosophy and capability of the top nursing executive.
4 The type of inservice training and education available.
5 The expectations of the clients and medical staff.
6 The demands of the administration.
7 The particular health care delivery system.
8 The community environment.

In general, the performance of head nurses is most influenced by the amount of authority delegated by the superior and by the amount of responsibility and accountability accepted by them as subordinates. Attitudes about time and risk factors, as well as feelings about subordinates and oneself greatly affect the amount of authority delegated (Volante 1976, pp. 66–67). Nurse executives tend *not* to delegate according to their perception of the following: delegation taking too much time; subordinates not having the necessary skills or not being trusted to perform competently; or preferring to do the job themselves rather than taking the blame for subordinates' actions. Because of these perceptions head nurses may underdelegate and overextend their responsibilities. When head nurses first assume the position, they may be continually asking for authorization from the supervisor or director when they are unsure of the jurisdiction and degree of positional power. Self-confidence and evidence of sound decision making will help to convince superiors that authority should be commensurate with responsibility. In the subordinate role, head nurses should take the initiative with higher management to participate in planning and policy-information and to give feedback. Being a subordinate does not mean being a passive recipient. Head nurses should become active participants in management even while learning and growing through interaction with other managers.

FUNCTIONING AS A HEAD NURSE

A head nurse can function without using managerial skills because a busy nursing unit almost runs itself as each need is met as it arises. Attending to countless details can consume so much time that none is left for planning, organizing, directing, coordinating, or controlling. Such an "unmanaged" unit delivers care that meets the lowest common denominator. The staff appear to be harried and frustrated; doctors are angry and demanding; and other hospital services avoid contact. Clients are uncomfortable, confused, and uncared for in a professional manner. In this situation, the head nurse is environmentally responsive—letting environment dictate his or her actions and responses. Instead, the head nurse could be environmentally effective—bringing about change in a demanding environment through the management process. (See page 19 for a further discussion of environmental responsiveness and effectiveness.)

DECISION MAKING

The primary tools of the management process are decision making, communication, and interpersonal relationships. Decision making is an integral part of all phases of the management process; it includes the definition of a problem, identification of alternatives, establishment of priorities, consideration of the constraints of each alternative, and deliberation about how to implement the solution to the problem. Nurses are educated to make decisions in an orderly way using the nursing process: assessment, planning, intervention, and evaluation. Other methods such as intuition, trial and error, reliance on tradition, rote memory, or deciding by default are insufficient and not conducive to arriving at good decisions.

Head nurses have the prerogative and authority to make many decisions that affect their units. By examining various ways of operating and the impact of the organizational system on their units, head nurses can discover that many different approaches contribute to efficiency, efficacy, improved motivation, and higher morale. The raw materials for decision making are the head nurse's designated responsibilities (including his or her skills, tasks, and functions) as well as the available resources (the head nurse's self-system, staff system, and other organization subsystems). It is the combination of responsibilities and resources that calls for creative decision making in such areas as staffing patterns, client assignments, workload, evaluation systems, teaching programs, rules and regulations, motivating factors, and budgets that pertain to the unit. Head nurses extend their influence in areas where they are not authorized to make decisions (for example, in hiring and firing staff nurses, devising a budget, and giving merit raises) by making recommendations substantiated by empirical evidence to higher authorities. These executives know that they must depend on head nurses to interpret their policies and implement their directives, and so there is reciprocity. By deciding what to tell whom, and in what way, the head nurse has a measure of control that goes beyond formal authority.

Decision-Making Styles

Besides the question of *what* decisions to make, there is the question of *how* to do so. There are several decision-making styles, but some are valued more highly than others. At present, the most highly valued style is democratic, participative decision making, which means that those who will be affected by a decision share in making it. Another style is autocratic decision making, in which managers who know that they will be held responsible make the decisions themselves. LaMonica and Finch (1977, p. 28) suggest that between these two poles—delegating a decision to others or making it oneself—there is a range of alternative styles. The use of a particular decision-making process should depend upon the situation. The variables to consider are the nurse-manager, nursing staff, clients, other resources, environment, goals, time, and urgency. Thus, sometimes those who are affected by a decision should participate in making it (even if they do not want to); at other times people should not participate in decision making (even if they want to). Two factors are important for the nurse-manager in choosing a particular style—the degree to which a problem is critical and the degree to which the solution requires acceptance and commitment. Five styles have been identified (LaMonica and Finch 1977, p. 21):

1 You make the decision yourself based on what you know.
2 You obtain information from others, and then decide yourself.
3 You share the problem with other individuals, and then decide yourself, but not necessarily taking their viewpoints into account.
4 You share the problem with a group, and then decide yourself, but not necessarily taking the group's viewpoint into account.
5 You share the problem with a group; the decision is a consensus of the group and is implemented as such.

Choosing style 1 does not automatically make a manager a "bad guy," and style 5 does not signify a "good guy," although this bias has been mentioned before. In making different decisions, nurse-managers should choose the appropriate style for a given problem. An experienced head nurse might use style 1 in deciding what supplies to order, whereas style 5 might be appropriate in deciding which nurse could attend the state nurses convention at the hospital's expense, or how to implement primary care nursing on the unit. Styles 2, 3, and 4 are utilized according to the particular individuals' and groups' problem-solving skills and the nurse-manager's group leadership abilities. These might be effective styles for making decisions about schedules, budgets, staffing, nursing care procedures, and client case study conferences. The advantages of varying the decision-making style to fit the situation include: the optimum use of human resources, the opportunity for subordinates to practice making decisions according to their perceived readiness, the increased commitment to implementation when the intentions of each style are made clear, and the personal and professional growth of the group when decisions are shared according to the needs and capabilities of each person.

COMMUNICATION AND RELATIONSHIP

A nurse-manager uses communication to implement the management process. Communication is a two-way process that includes a sender, a message, a receiver, and a feedback mechanism. When communication is clear and forthright with adequate feedback, work performance tends to match management's expectations. A major function of the head nurse is to give specific directions about what is expected in terms of the quantity and quality of work. The head nurse communicates about work to the nursing staff verbally and nonverbally by actions and attitudes. Examples of communications about work include: exhibiting behavior that is consistent with nursing philosophy and nursing practices; teaching new concepts and methods; coming to work on time and seldom being absent; acting as a role model in caring for clients; collaborating with other health professions; and reinforcing the expectations of performance by stating what is acceptable, what is required, and what is unacceptable.

Relationships are established through the communication process. Because communication has both a verbal and nonverbal component, subject to idiosyncratic interpretation, there is ample opportunity for misunderstanding, ambiguity, and conflict. The head nurse must establish good working relationships with the staff nurses, medical staff, clerical workers, the administrative superior, students, and the client family system. Also, as the interfacing person on the unit, the head nurse communicates with members of the various subsystems that provide supporting services such as dietary, pharmacy, medical records, x-ray, and social services. Interpersonal communication skills are essential for making these complex interactions purposeful and productive. To be an effective communicator, the head nurse must not only send a message so that it is clearly understood but also elicit feedback and hear *that* message's clear intent. Awareness of the physical and psychological barriers to good communication enables the nurse-manager to understand what barriers can be broken down. Physical barriers include space, distance, architecture, language, time, and lack of communication equipment. Psychological barriers are harder to deal with; they include selective inattention, inability to take suggestions from subordinates, poor self-concept, hearing only what one wants to hear, personality conflicts, attitudes, prejudices, and different cultural values.

The magnitude of the communication-relationship problem was vividly demonstrated at a workshop given by the author for first-line and middle management nurses. The participants were asked to list the conflicts or problems they had experienced in their organizations. After each nurse had independently complied a list and assigned each item a priority, the workshop leader had each person state the number 1 priority item, which was written on a blackboard. After each person had a turn, the procedure was repeated for priority number 2. On the third round duplications began to appear. Table 10-1 presents a list of the items mentioned, with check marks indicating the number of duplications for that item. More than half the items mentioned, counting the duplications pertain to communication and interpersonal relationships.

The head nurse who has recently been elevated from the ranks may have difficulty relating to his or her former peers as subordinates. Nurses who have a strong fear of being disliked or unpopular may hesitate to

Table 10-1   List of Problems and Conflicts*

	Apathy
	Interpersonal relationships
	Philosophy
✔	Clinical versus administrative responsibilities
	Work schedule
	Absenteeism
✔✔	Communication within the nursing department
	No voice in planning
✔	Caseload versus staff (client assignment)
	Caseload versus number of staff
✔	Inexperience
✔	Lack of self-confidence
	Lack of education
✔	Development of subordinates
✔	Rejection of authority by subordinates
	Reward system
	Communication between departments
	Control over referrals
✔	Learning motivation
	Bureaucracy
	Documentation
✔	Client needs versus staff rights
	Accountability
	"Patient care first"
	Authority
	Resistance to change
	Part-time versus full time
	Nurse-doctor communication
✔✔✔	Dual role
✔✔	Staff versus administration

✔ = Duplication of response
* = These items are listed at random.

communicate orders and difficult decisions. For instance, one head nurse rationalized that because the turnover rate was very low on her unit (all nurses had worked there from three to eight years), she could overlook the high absenteeism of three nurses rather than confront them and risk losing their good will. However, it would have been better to call the absenteeism to their attention, explicitly describe the consequences if it should continue, and follow through with the stipulated disciplinary action, or reward a change in behavior. A helpful way to facilitate this is the management practice of contracting between superior and subordinate (see Chapter 11). Other methods to clarify roles and mixed messages are group conferences, individual performance appraisal sessions, on-the-spot observation and confrontation, nursing rounds, and generally maintaining a profile of high visibility and approachability.

The head nurse's relationships with the medical staff and attending physicians can run the gamut from overt hostility to collaborative team work. Individual personalities and socialization of sexual and professional roles are probably the major determinant of the quality of the nurse-doctor relationship. The head nurse, more so than a staff nurse, can deal from a position of strength in establishing a relationship with a doctor. First of all, the unit is clearly defined as the head nurse's territory; the medical staff come and go, while the nurse remains on the unit. Both doctor and head nurse assume 24-hour responsibility for clients and are accountable in a clearly defined way. Also, both the doctor and head nurse have to rely on others (mostly the staff nurses) to carry out their directives for medical and nursing care. This does not mean that on occasion the head nurse will not be blamed by the doctor if "something goes wrong" with the client, or the family complains to the doctor. However, most doctors respect and cooperate with the head nurse who demonstrates clinical competency, professional judgment, and the ability to collaborate with mutual trust. At times, the head nurse may act as liaison between the medical staff with whom he or she has good rapport and the nursing staff.

Maintaining a good working relationship with the administration is another important and necessary aspect of the head nurse's work. Frequently the value systems of the nurse and the administrator collide when there is a conflict of interest, such as when the delivery system of nursing care must be balanced with cost and efficiency. The following example typifies this dilemma:

> A hospital administrator determined that it would cost less to use a three-shift cycle for the nursing staff on the operating-recovery rooms unit than to continue with the on-call system that had existed for many years. He directed the head nurse on the unit to figure out how to institute his plan without changing the present staff. After much deliberation and some discussion with her staff, the head nurse drew up a schedule for three shifts. She had secured the cooperation of several staff members who would be permanently assigned to evenings and nights, provided they had most weekends off. Her plan included an elaborate system for rotating duties so that all nurses had a fair share. However, to accomplish her plan she needed four more nurses.
>
> The administrator refused to allow four nurses to be added, but insisted that the head nurse institute her plan anyway. The plan had to be modified so that all nurses rotated shifts and worked two out of three weekends to provide coverage.
>
> Within three weeks, seven nurses quit and absenteeism was very high. Supervisory personnel were compelled to fill in because the new nurses on the unit and the "floaters" were not experienced enough for safe practice in the OR. Two weeks later, the administrator rescinded the order and reinstituted the old on-call system.

This example illustrates many points about communication break-down, the need for planned change, and the problems created by unquestioned values. The administrator saw the head nurse's request for more nurses as an unnecessary luxury. From his point of view, so long as the "business" of the operating room continued without mishap, he did not need to question the means. If the head nurse and nursing supervisors had enlisted the doctors in their cause and prevented the operating room from functioning by refusing to fill in, the outcome might have been different.

The head nurse is the person who interfaces with all the other departments and divisions in the organization; this is the coordinating function of management. In today's hospital organization, coordinating takes much more of the head nurse's time than formerly when being head nurse meant that one person performed *all* services for the client. The system becomes even more complex by increased demands for highly specialized services as well as the trend toward hotel-like accommodations. When the system breaks down as, for example, when meal trays do not arrive as ordered, clients go to the operating room late, or the maintenance engineer cannot be located to fix a leaky faucet, the head nurse takes the blame. Keeping the system operating efficiently is a job that demands persuasiveness, patience, and ingenuity.

The client and the family are subsystems that require close attention and consideration as prime consumers of nursing care and the *raison d'être* for the health care organization. As family care nursing becomes a reality, the head nurse must assume some responsibilities for "customer relations." The head nurse attempts to maintain a relationship with the client, and especially the family, in such a way that their objectives can be harmonized with those of the organization. At times, the head nurse acts as the organization's advocate—explaining policies, orienting the family to the facility, offering its services, and giving information. This is especially important when the client and family first arrive on the unit. In initiating a relationship, the head nurse sets the tone for future meetings and lends authority to discussions about policies and the proposed treatment regimen. Whenever the client and family's needs do not fit the normal pattern, the head nurse works as the client's advocate to bend the rules or shape the policy to provide greater satisfaction. The nurse-manager draws on the resources at his or her disposal in a way that is useful to the family and supportive of the staff.

Longest (1976, pp. 181–182) suggests how to improve communication skills within the organization:

1 Have a clear idea of what you want to say before you communicate it.
2 Look at the real meaning of each communication.

3 Consider the total environmental system whenever you communicate.

4 Consult with others when planning a communication.

5 Consider both the verbal and the nonverbal message of your communication.

6 Look for opportunities to convey positive messages and values.

7 Ask for feedback to your communication.

8 Do not postpone difficult or negative communications.

9 Be consistent in what you say and do.

10 Be a good listener.

The head nurse who consciously implements the management process through effective decision making and communication makes an impact on the organization, brings order out of chaos, and provides a climate that fosters professional growth and personal satisfaction among the staff members.

SUMMARY

All nurses are managers because the practice of nursing parallels the practice of management. The head nurse is a first-line manager who occupies a position in the organizational hierarchy. Nurses are frequently promoted because of their excellent clinical skills. However, leadership skills and a background in management theory are equally important to be a successful and effective nurse-manager.

Head nurses have difficulty reconciling the dual role implied in *nurse-manager*—one who must report to two authorities. Without preparatory education, head nurses have difficulty handling clinical and managerial responsibilities, particularly if they have not internalized the role of manager. Successful performance as a head nurse depends upon the amount of authority delegated by the nursing executive, as well as the amount of responsibility and accountability accepted by the head nurse as subordinate.

Decision making and communication are the principal tools used by the head nurse in the management process. The most useful decision-making style is one that fits the given situation. Communication and the establishment of relationships with the nursing staff, medical staff, administration, other support subsystems, and the client and family are discussed from the head nurse's perspective.

REFERENCES

Galloway, B. T. 1974. The nurse as a professional manager. *Hospitals, J.A.H.A.* 48 (November 1):89,92,94.

Ganong, Joan M.; and Ganong, Warren L. 1976. *Nursing management.* German-town, Md.: Aspen Systems.

——. 1975. Are head nurses obsolete? *Journal of Nursing Administration* 5,9:16–18.

LaMonica, Elaine; and Finch, Frederic E. 1977. Managerial decision making. *Journal of Nursing Administration* 7,3:20–28.

Longest, Beaufort B., Jr. 1976. *Management practices for the health profes-sional.* Reston, Va.: Reston Publishing.

Plachy, Roger J. 1976. Head nurses: less griping, more action. *Journal of Nursing Administration* 6,1:39–41.

Shea, Carole A. 1978. *Management in nursing: putting the process to work.* Workshop presented at Downstate Medical Center, Brooklyn, New York.

Sills, Grayce M. 1976. Nursing, medicine, and hospital administration. *American Journal of Nursing* 76,9:1432–1434.

Stevens, Barbara J. 1975. *The nurse as executive.* Wakefield, Mass.: Contempo-rary.

Volante, Elena M. 1976. Mastering the managerial skill of delegation. *In Man-agement for nurses,* ed. Sandra Stone et al. St. Louis: Mosby, pp. 65–69.

SUGGESTED READINGS

Barrett, Jean; Gessner, Barbard A.; Phelps, Charlene. 1975. *The head nurse,* 3rd ed. New York: Appleton-Century-Crofts.

Douglass, Laura Mae; and Bevis, Em Olivia. 1974. *Nursing leadership in action.* St. Louis: Mosby.

Eckrahl, Virginia R. 1976. On-the-job management training. *Journal of Nursing Administration* 6,2:38–40.

Kilpack, Virginia. 1976. The head nurse creates a new order for clinical learning. *Journal of Nursing Administration* 6,10:41–46.

Mealy, Sharon; et al. 1977. Shared leadership—no head nurse! *Nursing Adminis-tration Quarterly* 1,1:81–93.

Miller, Patricia. 1976. Open minds to new ideas! an injunction for nursing leaders. *Journal of Nursing Administration* 6,4:18–22.

Chapter 11

Managing by Contract

John M. Oakes

OBJECTIVES

After studying this chapter, the learner will:

- Define dualism in management of a health care system
- Define performance contracting
- Explain the relationship between management by objectives and performance contracting
- List the steps in writing a performance contract
- Discuss the link between contracting and the annual performance appraisal

SERVICE ORGANIZATIONS

The task of managing within a system that has a nonprofit, service orientation presents unique problems and opportunities that are seldom addressed in management literature. Newman and Warren (1977, p. 101) feel that these unique characteristics call for special management attention; they list six characteristics of nonprofit organizations:

1   The service provided is usually intangible, and its quality is hard to measure—often there are multiple objectives.
2   Consumer influence is weak; usually the organization has a local monopoly position within the community.
3   The employees are usually committed primarily to their professions and secondarily to their organization.
4   The major resource contributors intrude upon internal management, notably governmental agencies or large benefactors.
5   The availability of performance rewards is limited. Salary and promotion are often based on qualifications or seniority. When coupled with number 1 above, demotion or dismissal for cause can be difficult.
6   Charismatic leaders or institutional "mystique" are significant means for resolving conflict within the organization.

Virtually all of these characteristics are relevant to health care delivery systems. The dualism caused by two formal management subsystems—one based upon the authority of position (as represented by the administrative hierarchy) and the other based upon specialization and professional knowledge (as represented by practitioners of all types)—creates the need for an integrated matrix-management process (see pages 32–35) that is both diffuse and complex. This type of system can frustrate even the most competent manager.

Although the health care management process may be complex, the major goals and underlying values of the system are reasonably clear. The overriding objective is to satisfy the needs of the consumer for care and treatment; this "mystique" unifies the varying objectives of the administrative staff, nurses, medical staff, clients, trustees, and others. It is this mystique, when it must face the realities imposed by economics, medical technology, and the management dualism mentioned above, that can cause frustration and role conflict for nurses who must operate as managers within the system.

Management by contracting, properly implemented, suggests itself as an appropriate method to achieve explicit understanding and joint agreement on responsibilities shared with superiors, subordinates, peers, or clients. It also permits objective performance evaluation. Thus, it can provide a partial solution to some of the recurrent management problems that nurses are experiencing in hospitals.

WHAT IS PERFORMANCE CONTRACTING?

A contract is an agreement between two parties to do or not to do a particular task or series of tasks. Typically, contracts specify the duties to be performed, the order in which they will be performed, the person who is responsible for performing them, and what rights or responsibilities each side has by virtue of entering into the contract.

Contracts need not be written. Often in business, particularly in finance, oral contracts are the rule rather than the exception. Each day in New York and London, hundreds of millions of dollars change hands in very complex currency and commodity transactions. It is rare for these oral contracts to be supported by written signed agreements. It is rarer still to have a dispute between the contracting parties. Two necessary preconditions to these oral contracts are an unusual degree of mutual trust and long experience with a basically repetitive transaction structure. Oral contracts can probably work effectively without one of these preconditions, but not both. For managers who wish to apply the concept of contracting in a hospital setting, written contracts will probably be preferred. Some advantages of a written contract are:

1 It provides certainty (given the constraints of language) since there is no need to rely on the memories of the contracting parties, which may become unreliable if there is a dispute.

2 It can specify the binding time deadlines which protect both sides against change without prior notice.

3 It explicitly establishes minimum quality standards for the delivery of goods or services.

4 It provides clear-cut procedures for solving disputes between the contracting parties.

5 It specifies the method, form, and time of payment for the contracted good or service; or the procedures for withholding payment; or the penalties in case of nondelivery or delivery of a low quality product.

Due to the multiple roles of a nurse in a hospital, often many of his or her total job responsibilities are not explicitly stated. The written job description usually does not provide a clear idea of the nurse-manager's expectations for his or her performance, even when it lists a complete range of required tasks. Unstated expectations will not help the nurse to be autonomous; rather, they tend to leave him or her frustrated, in the dark, and unable to perceive the important tasks of what judgment criteria the nurse-manager will use to evaluate specific performance.

The manager usually feels the need to "lay out the ground rules" to a new subordinate and does so, but often balks at frank, mutual discussion of exactly what will be expected from his or her subordinates; this happens either because the job requirements or the performance standards are unclear to the manager, or because the manager does not have the time, training, or inclination to be specific. Sometimes the manager's resistance may stem from a normal reluctance to criticize subordinates and a belief that attempts to change what has been done previously may imply

criticism of the earlier performance. These are typical cases where contracting will help to clarify complex and unspecific job situations.

In using performance contracting, the subordinate and manager
would first identify mutually acceptable areas for performance and the
minimum acceptable performance standard for each area. The process of
achieving agreement may be as important to them as is the delineation of
areas and standards, since it provides the opportunity for both to communicate their perception of and expectations for their work relationships.

When they decide to formalize their understandings in a contract,
there is no thought of exchanging money for service. The manager is not
"employing" the subordinate; rather, they are establishing explicit standards of performance and mutual responsibility for achieving that performance standard. The unique features of the process are:

1   The participants set the objectives.
2   It provides for periodic review of the contract in terms of performance versus expectations and the continued relevance of the contracted
areas in view of changing work requirements.
3   It separates annual performance evaluation from progress toward
fulfilling the contract. Therefore, results that are below standard can be
viewed positively (as requiring problem diagnosis and solution) instead of
negatively (as failures to be blamed on an accountable manager).
4   It links performance evaluation to the future development needs
of the subordinate; an effort is made to plan for building skills that will be
used during the next contracting period.

HOW DOES CONTRACTING "FIT" IN THE MANAGEMENT PROCESS?

Contracting can be viewed as the formalization of an implicit part of the
management process (planning, organizing, directing, coordinating, and
controlling). In most organizations, the subordinate provides input for the
manager's planning and organizing efforts. This input usually takes the
form of suggestions as to overall direction or levels of achievement that
the subordinate feels represent possible performance. Although this process can be initiated by either side, the manager is seldom obliged to use
this input or to explain why it was not used. The subordinate's involvement in coordinating, directing, and controlling is more tangential, and it
is usually the result of his or her output or actual performance, which
tends to modify the coordinating, directing, and controlling activities of
the manager who gives feedback on the subordinate's activities.

Contracting, then, formalizes the input process between manager and
subordinate. It also helps to set standards for the subordinate's output. It

embodies the concept that management must be a participative process if it is to be successful. This means that the subordinate's participative role in structuring what is to be done, in deciding how best to accomplish it, and in establishing standards for judging what is accomplished is at least equal to that of the manager.

WHAT IS MBO?

This process of explicitly setting objectives is at the core of one of the most widely discussed and analyzed management methods, that is, management by objectives (MBO). The term *management by objectives* was first used by Peter Drucker in 1954. Drucker saw MBO as a method for improving managerial motivation since, at its best, MBO is able to integrate an organization's goals with the individual manager's need to be an effective contributor and to develop personally (Humble 1973, p. 4). The fundamental assumption of MBO is that the organization can be described as a hierarchy of goals, and that management's task is to formulate objectives that will achieve them and to organize activities accordingly. It is also assumed that specific performance criteria for individuals or organizations within the system can be integrated with the objective-setting process. Thus, managers and subordinates try to achieve commitment to both the criteria and the objective-setting process. Levinson (1970, p. 125) speaks of MBO as a way of permitting the manager to determine his objectives from a range of potential options. Once chosen, the MBO process assumes that the manager will: (1) work hard to achieve them, (2) be motivated by peers and subordinates because of the explicit commitment, and (3) be responsible to the organization for doing so. Reddin (1970, pp. 13–14) indicated that, while the MBO process can vary among organizations and theorists, it usually contains the following elements:

1   Establishment of objectives for managerial positions. It must be decided what the manager is to achieve, and specific targets for performance must be set.
2   Use of joint objective setting. The superior and the subordinate participate in setting objectives. Minimally, the subordinate attends the meeting where objectives are announced and has a right to be heard. Maximally, the subordinate initiates the objective-setting process.
3   Linking of objectives. Objectives cannot be set in a vacuum; in most systems, one manager's objectives require complementary objectives for other groups. For example, head nurses have the objective to make sure that dietary plans for patients are followed. This requires that the dietician have the objective of preparing meals in accordance with the dietary plans. Linking is usually noticed by its absence—when there is very loud feedback.

4 Emphasis on measurement and control. All MBO systems stress the necessity of being able to measure results. Without measurement, attainment of the objective cannot be known. Without control, objectives are simply predictions.

5 Establishment of review and recycle systems. All MBO systems have a periodic review of progress. During these reviews, attempts are made to measure progress toward objectives, remove impediments to their achievement, or revise the objectives in view of the tentative results. This review always includes the manager and subordinate.

All of this may be seen as the embodiment of good management, that is, effective goal setting; genuine participation; and a constructive, non-threatening performance orientation. Yet, MBO is not management; it is a reliance on a formal mechanism to improve motivation and performance (DeFee 1977, p. 39). Performance contracting is one of the tools used within the MBO context to formalize the implicit understandings between subordinate and manager.

WRITING THE CONTRACT

Before writing a sample contract, one must note the definitions of the terms that will be used. These concepts appear in many texts under a variety of names.

Performance area. The general output requirements of a managerial position. These can range from areas that are shared with many peers to job-specific or individual-specific areas.

Objectives. The specific tasks to be accomplished in each performance area.

Performance standard. The specific level of required output and the measurement criteria for that objective. These criteria should be as time-specific and measurable as possible.

Progress review. A periodic evaluation meeting between manager and subordinate (possibly on a quarterly basis) where they both review progress toward completion of the objectives.

Development action plan. A specific plan written by the manager (usually following an annual performance appraisal) in which he or she outlines the process by which the subordinate will develop critical skills required by the job or, if the subordinate's performance is noticeably above standard, future suitable assignment options.

The process of writing the contract entails a number of steps, most of which must be jointly agreed to by the manager and the subordinate. Which person actually initiates each step is not so important as achieving agreement at each stage. Table 11-1 lists the steps to be followed in writing a contract:

Table 11-1 Steps in Writing a Performance Contract

---

1 Determine the relevant performance areas.

2 Set the objectives to be met in each performance area.

3 Structure the performance standards for each objective.

4 Establish the relative importance of different performance areas.

5 Decide upon the frequency and content of progress reviews.

6 Outline the manager's responsibility to provide a development action plan at the conclusion of the contract.

STEP 1: DEFINE THE PERFORMANCE AREAS

While every managerial position has performance areas, sometimes they may not be written in the job description or even known to workers. Performance areas are those that define the true function of the position. For most positions there are both general and specific performance areas. For example, a clinical specialist's general performance areas include (Reddin 1970, p. 40):

1 Professional competence.
2 Consultation in area of competence.
3 Acceptance of the specialist's advice.
4 Improvement due to acceptance of the advice.

As part of the process of determining relevant performance areas, the nurse-manager and the superior try to define the major areas of interface or responsibility for clients, subordinates, superiors, physicians, and self.

Questions such as the following may help to delineate performance areas: (1) What specific tasks does the nurse-manager perform for each group? (2) What specific tasks should be performed? (3) Which of those tasks are significant, considering the nurse-manager's continuing responsibilities? and (4) Which tasks are unique to the nurse-manager?

Since this is a participative process, management should try to listen as much as possible and ask questions to draw out the subordinate manager's opinions such as: "What are your plans? How can I help?" or "What can you do for the hospital that I haven't given you a chance to do?" The performance areas should be described in neutral terms, typically using from one to four words, for example: "To provide care." (There should be no descriptions of performance quality such as: "To provide *efficient* care.") Finally, although there is some dispute on this point in the literature, it is not necessary to detail every area of specific responsibility; the idea is simply to pinpoint the significant areas for which the nurse-manager will be accountable.

STEP 2: SET THE OBJECTIVES TO BE MET IN EACH PERFORMANCE AREA

The objectives should be quite specific statements about what is to be accomplished in each performance area. Depending upon the position, they can be measured by: time (how soon), quantity (how many), quality (how well) or cost (how much). Del Bueno (1977, p. 21) differentiates between doing a thing right and doing the right thing. The former refers to technical competence, that is, performing a task at the minimum acceptable standard. Such tasks ought to be measured by performance checklists and not viewed as objectives to be included in a performance contract. Appropriate contracting objectives are those behaviors that could be called "doing the right thing," since making a clinical judgment requires a mixture of training, observation, and evaluation.

STEP 3: STRUCTURE THE PERFORMANCE STANDARDS

This answers the question "What *really* constitutes satisfactory performance?" As part of this process, it is important for the subordinate and manager to try to agree on the measurement criteria for each performance objective. These should be as precise as possible, with little room for subjective interpretation. Three aspects must be covered:

1 Measurement criteria: "What will we look at?"
2 Measurement method: "How will we look at it?"
3 Measurement interpretation: "What does it mean?"

Every effort should be made to try to reach an agreement on performance standards. Sometimes, however, this proves to be impossible; disagreement is most frequent in the area of interpretation. In those cases, the manager's interpretation must prevail. This is a ground rule for all phases of contracting to which the subordinate must agree in advance. Occasionally the standard is not directly quantifiable: "Ensure clear communication with physician" is an objective for which the performance standard is no substitute for the acutal performance. "No negative feedback" (see Table 11-2) does not mean that the nurse communicated clearly; it is simply the best effort at a quantifiable approximation of the performance.

STEP 4: ESTABLISH THE RELATIVE IMPORTANCE OF DIFFERENT PERFORMANCE AREAS

Clearly all performance areas are not of equal importance. During any given period the manager may want to focus on certain aspects of the job while deemphasizing others. The relative ranking should be determined after the performance standards have been set so that the subordinate does not already have a stake in making the primary objectives either too easy or too difficult to measure depending upon his or her perception of their achievability.

STEP 5: DECIDE UPON THE FREQUENCY AND CONTENT OF PROGRESS REVIEWS

The progress review is an essential element in the participative process of tracking performance toward objectives. The manager and subordinate should agree in advance as to how often reviews should take place. The frequency can vary depending upon the nature of the objectives: Routinized objectives can be managed on an exception basis, that is, evaluated and discussed when something goes wrong. Ongoing programs that are very complex might be reviewed monthly or whenever a milestone is passed. Other objectives may require periodic attention and therefore should be reviewed monthly or quarterly. In most cases the subordinate will benefit from frequent coaching and progress reviews of a generalized nature; most theorists believe that there should be at least four joint meetings each year (quarterly reviews). Both parties should be jointly responsible for initiating the periodic reviews.

STEP 6: OUTLINE A DEVELOPMENT ACTION PLAN

The manager should prepare the development action plan. As a counselor or coach, therefore, the manager attempts to build the skills that the subordinate will need in order to be effective in the future. The plan should be written, signed by both, and attached to the subordinate's performance appraisal; it should detail the specific steps (training, job experience, continuing education) that the manager thinks are required to keep or make the subordinate fully qualified with respect to the skills required by the position.

Any outline of what can or should be achieved in contract form carries with it a series of implicit assumptions that are critical to the subordinate's ability to perform in accordance with the contract. Because these assumptions can change, it is useful to list the major ones somewhere in the body of the contract; examples of these assumptions include: staff levels, budget, generalized mission, and existing training requirements.

A SAMPLE CONTRACT

Table 11-2 shows a completed contract between a head nurse and supervisor. It outlines five performance areas and twenty objectives, together

Table 11-2 Sample Performance Contract

The following was drawn up at several performance planning discussions between Nancy White, Head Nurse, 3 West; and Ima Ogre, Nursing Supervisor; Fallen Pines Hospital. The performance areas for which Nancy White will be responsible during 1980 and the relevant standard of performance required to achieve a fully satisfactory rating on her performance appraisal have been agreed upon jointly:

Performance areas	Performance standards
1 Client care:	
a Plan nursing care	Care is safe, economical, efficient, and meets relevant standards, for example JCAH and ANA
b Plan and assist in health teaching of client	Client demonstrates comprehension and performs satisfactorily
c See to it that quality care is given to each client	Care plan documentation, other records, and feedback indicate standards are met
d Use the care plan developed in *(a)* to assist in resolving client problems	Care plan documentation indicates sustaining action on problems and progress toward discharge
e Give direct care to clients as required	Same as *(c)* above
f Act as liaison between client, physician, and family	Client and family understand and can carry out physician's directions; feedback is provided to physician
2 Medical staff:	
a See that the doctor's orders are carried out	Orders are carried out promptly and accurately
b Act as liaison between physician and client care team	Communications, as documented and used on care plan, are clear
c Ensure clear communication with physician	No documented errors; no negative feedback
3 Subordinate staff:	
a Act as leader, problem-solver, and model	Appropriate example set; staff feedback indicates feeling of acceptance of role model
b Delegate responsibility where required	Staff and client's needs are met; action is not held up unnecessarily pending Head Nurse's decisions on routine matters
c Assure adequate staffing	Personnel are assigned for optimum utilization and adequate coverage
d Promote staff-member training and development	Evidence of participation in continuing education programs
e Assist in development and usage of nursing care plans	Care plans are current and appropriate on daily basis
f Plan for future of subordinates	Staff understands "where they stand" and "where they are going"

Table 11-2 Sample Performance Contract (continued)

4 Other organizational components:

a Promote cooperation across departments	Perceived good working relationships; no negative feedback
b Coordinate responses to proposed policy changes	Floor or area provides reasoned input in advance to proposed policies

5 Self:

a Keep technical skills up-to-date	Technical job competence continues to meet established performance standards
b Develop new skills	Broadened base of skills provide growth in overall job competency
c Improve or maintain sense of satisfaction with job	Perceived sense of well-being

Ms. White's primary focus will be in performance areas 1 and 3, which will account for 70 percent of her rating, with areas 2, 4, and 5 weighted equally.

We have agreed that progress toward the above performance standards will be reviewed frequently, at least once each quarter. At that time, we may add, modify, or eliminate elements in either the Performance Areas or Performance Standards. We further agree that we are jointly responsible for initiating the progress review meetings. We both understand and agree that Ms. White's annual performance appraisal will be based solely upon the above, including modifications (if any), and not on other extraneous measures. We recognize that it will be Ms. Ogre's responsibility, subsequent to the performance appraisal, to recommend a development action plan for Ms. White for the following year, including (if necessary) action to develop critical skills or, if her performance is noticeably above standard, future suitable assignment options.

This contract is based upon a variety of implicit assumptions about Ms. White's working environment, including the existing budget, staffing levels, and generalized mission of 3 West.

Nancy White	Ima Ogre
Head Nurse	Nursing Supervisor

*Adapted from Ganong, Joan M.; and Warren L. Ganong, *Nursing Management.* Germantown, Md.: Aspen Systems, 1976, pp. 305–307.

with the associated performance standards for each. This example is meant to illustrate the contracting process and so it does not deal with either the measurement of technical skills or the extended range of responsibilities of most head nurses.

THE CONTRACT AND THE PERFORMANCE APPRAISAL

After the performance contract has been written and largely fulfilled, the subordinate may ask, "How will this contract work for me?" The sample contract (Table 11-2) specified that the manager would not use external, subjective criteria to evaluate the subordinate. In fact, if the periodic progress reviews are carried out as planned, nothing in the performance appraisal could come as a surprise to the subordinate. In many texts, the MBO process does not even call for a discrete performance evaluation since such evaluation is continuous and the MBO process emphasizes improving for the future (Patz 1975, p. 79). Most performance appraisals have a historical orientation, linking past behavior with past results. However, most organizations that utilize MBO still have some sort of performance appraisal system. Regardless of what kind of appraisal system is used, the completed performance contract can enable the subordinate and manager to deal with virtually any appraisal system as objectively as it is humanly possible.

Notwithstanding the safeguards suggested above, it is important to understand the dichotomy in appraisal objectives. Winstanley (1972, p. 60) says that the purpose of the appraisal dictates the criteria, method, and type of feedback to be employed. The organization must decide whether to use the appraisal to determine and justify salary increases or to develop people, that is, to sharpen and develop their skills. Cummings and Schwab (1973, p. 5) show that the reward approach places the manager in a judgmental role, whereas the developmental approach places the manager in a counseling role. The position of the subordinate is also significantly affected. When the manager is judgmental, the subordinate is either passive or reactive if he or she must defend past actions. When the manager is acting as a counselor, the subordinate is actively learning. Winstanley (p. 60) suggests that a reward orientation requires results-oriented criteria whereas a development orientation requires personal, means-oriented criteria. Many theorists have commented on this dualism, in which managers must use either means-oriented criteria in pay decisions or results-oriented criteria for development. In the first case the incentive relationship is weakened. In the second case, the relevance of the results to improving skills is often not too explicit. If managers are asked to fill a dual role, they are placed in an impossible situation where they cannot conduct an effective, successful appraisal (McGregor 1972, p. 138).

The performance contract tries to eliminate this dichotomy by emphasizing the developmental aspects of performance; the manager must produce a development action plan for the subordinate. Schlesinger (1976, p. 274) points out that the subordinate has three options for dealing with performance data:

1 The data can be ignored.
2 They can be filed in the subordinate's memory bank, where they will be occasionally remembered and reacted to.
3 They can be studied and used to make positive behavioral changes.

The manager who initiates a development action plan assumes that the subordinate wants to make positive behavioral changes and that the data will be meaningful and valid. Then the manager and subordinate have a discussion, in which the latter may ask the following questions:

1 Is my behavior worth changing in this area? (What's in it for me? For example, career advancement, better relationship with the manager.)
2 How should I change? The desired change must be well defined.
3 How will I change? Should outside courses, inservice training, more exposure to the manager, or a combination be used?
4 When should it be done? Since procrastination is a human trait, a timetable is a useful tool.
5 How will I know when it's done? The subordinate needs feedback and should be told in advance exactly what kind will be used.

After these questions have been answered and the plan formalized, progress toward its achievement should be made part of the periodic progress review. The development action plan should be included under the umbrella of the performance appraisal and be fed back into the performance contract for the next period.

Efforts such as these that attempt to improve the chances that good performance will be rewarded and that poor performance corrected help to improve morale, motivation, and thereby performance. According to McGregor (1972, p. 138), the front-loaded implementation time required from managers is considerably more with systems that try to modify behavior (such as performance contracting). Management's reaction to this real cost will vary from strongly positive to strongly negative. One indicator of management's sensitivity to the importance of developing its human resources will be its commitment to such a process.

CONTRACTING TO EFFECT CHANGE

The manager is the ultimate change agent within any system (Kast and Rosenzweig 1974, p. 578); thus, change can arise from any adjustments initiated by the manager in leadership style, approaches to planning, or controlling. Equally important, managers may react to suggestions from subordinates, consultants, or others inside or outside the system. Contracting is a way to focus on problems that require change and to provide the required communication and evaluation structure between the manager and subordinate to make sure that, once decided, change can be implemented. The contracting process also provides for feedback—criticism, evaluation, and followup of newly instituted changes.

SUMMARY

The dualism of the two formal management subsystems operating within the hospital creates a diffuse and complex system that often leaves critical objectives unstated, and the relevant standards of performance difficult to perceive. The process of performance contracting can help to make these objectives and standards explicit, thereby reducing tension between the manager and subordinate, particularly if they can reach a joint agreement via a participative objective-setting process. Contracting is one way to formalize certain steps in the management by objectives process, since it defines the performance areas, objectives, and performance standards that are integral components of most MBO systems. Contracting can help managers avoid the dilemma of choosing between the role of judge or counselor, which is dictated by the dual purpose of most performance appraisal systems; contracting tends to focus on a developmental rather than a judgmental role.

Since contracting is a future-oriented, behavior-modification process that tries to develop subordinates' abilities while meeting the organization's objectives, it can be a significant asset to responsible managers.

REFERENCES

Cummings, L. L.; and Schwab, Donald P. 1973. *Performance in organizations.* Glenview, Ill.: Scott, Foresman.

DeFee, Dallas T. 1977. Management by objectives: when and how does it work? *Personnel Journal* 56,1:37–39.

del Bueno, Dorothy J. 1977. Performance evaluation: when all is said and done, more is said than done. *Journal of Nursing Administration* 12,10:21–23.

Ganong, Joan; and Ganong, Warren. 1976. *Nursing management.* Germantown, Md.: Aspen Systems.

Humble, John W. 1973. *How to manage by objectives*. London: AMACOM.

Kast, Fremont E.; Rosenzweig, James W. 1974. *Organization management*. New York: McGraw-Hill.

Levinson, Harry. 1970. Management by whose objectives? *Harvard Business Review* 48,4:125.

McGregor, Douglas. 1972. An uneasy look at performance appraisal. *Harvard Business Review* 50,5:133– 138.

Newman, William H.; and Warren, E. Kirby. 1977. *The process of management*. Englewood Cliffs, N.J.: Prentice-Hall.

Patz, Alan L. 1975. Performance appraisal: useful but still resisted. *Harvard Business Review* 53,3:74–80.

Reddin, W. J. 1971. *Effective management by objectives*. New York: McGraw-Hill.

Schlesinger, Len. 1976. Performance improvement: the missing element. *Personnel Journal* 55,6:274–275.

Winstanley, N. B. 1972. Performance appraisal: another pollution problem? *The Conference Board Record* (September): 59–63.

SUGGESTED READINGS

Carroll, Archie B.; and Anthony, Ted F. 1976. An overview of the supervisor's job. *Personnel Journal* 55,5:228–231,249.

Drucker, Peter. 1974. *Management: tasks, responsibilities, practices*. New York: Harper and Row.

Lundberg, Craig C.; and Sproule, Robert E. 1968. Readiness for management development: an exploratory note. *California Management Review* 10 (Summer):73–80.

Meyer, Herbert H.; Kay, Emanuel; and French, John R. P., Jr. 1971. Split roles in performance appraisal. *Harvard Business Review* 49,2:123–129.

Odiorne, George. 1965. *Management by objectives*. New York: Pitman.

Rieder, George A. 1973. Performance review—a mixed bag. *Harvard Business Review* 51,4:61–67.

Chapter 12

The Nurse as Client Advocate

Shelley Van Kempen

OBJECTIVES

After studying this chapter, the learner will:

- Define advocacy
- Describe the sociohistorical development of the advocacy role
- List ways in which a nurse may function as a client advocate
- List advantages and disadvantages of the advocate role

DEFINITION OF ADVOCACY

An advocate is one who defends or intervenes on behalf of another. A nurse is an advocate when he or she acts for and in the interest of the client's welfare. This definition sounds relatively simple, but it raises several issues. For example, who decides what action will or will not benefit the client? If several choices are available, who chooses? Who decides what alternatives will be considered? The basic issue in advocacy, and perhaps nursing itself, is who will be in charge of the client's well-being. Conceivably, using the above definition, a nurse could decide that a client needs an advocate or defender, select an outcome for one of the client's problems, and initiate measures to produce that outcome—but without consulting the client! The fallacy of such an approach is demonstrated in a 1972 study (Dodge 1972, pp. 1852–1854) in which there was a great discrepancy between what the nurses felt clients *should* be told and what the clients *wanted* to be told. Of necessity, then, the definition of advocacy in nursing needs to be expanded. On the question of who will be in charge of the client's well-being, the answer must be the client. The client's autonomy must be clear in any definition of advocacy.

Consider the kinds of situations where a client might require an advocate, a defender, or an intercessor:

1 The client has a health care problem that is not understood or remains unsolved despite repeated interventions.
2 The client does not understand or is unaware of his or her rights as a consumer of health care.
3 The client does not know what to expect in the way of care from the health care system.
4 The client does not know who is able or willing to help solve his or her problem(s).
5 The client is thwarted by the complex rules of a bureaucratic system.
6 The client receives inadequate, unsafe, or indifferent care.

All of these examples have one thing in common: because of a lack of knowledge about health care and the health care system, the client is *powerless* to make it work for him or her. Most people need to control events that affect them, and any loss of that control—the ability to decide what will happen—creates distress. The goal of advocacy is to put power back into the hands of the health care consumer.

An advocate is one who increases the client's autonomy and self-determination. Specific nurse-advocate behaviors would include:

1 Increasing the clients' knowledge about their health problems so that they are able to make appropriate choices.
2 Informing clients about their rights as health care consumers and seeing that these rights are upheld.
3 Making resources available to meet clients' needs and then allowing them to select which ones they will use.
4 Keeping communication among client-family-doctor-nurse open and clear in order to prevent misunderstandings.

5 Making the health care system more responsive and sensitive to clients by educating other health professionals and serving as a role model.

(Case examples of these behaviors will be given later in the chapter.) Anyone who has worked in a bureaucratic system knows how easily the efficient operation (goals) of the organization can become antithetical to the needs of clients. In a sense, then, a client advocate "trouble shoots," looking for injustices and inadequacies within the health care system.

SOCIOHISTORICAL DEVELOPMENT OF THE ADVOCACY ROLE

Implementation of the advocacy role and increased client autonomy will lead to a shift in the traditional relationship between health care providers and consumers. Basically a transfer of knowledge is required and the role of the advocate is to facilitate this transfer.

The traditional provider-consumer model has health professionals firmly in control of the clients' decision making because of their special knowledge and experience. Professionals are expected to share their knowledge on demand, but they maintain control over how much and to whom they disseminate this knowledge. Friedson (1974, p. 28) writes that it is the *exclusiveness* of professionals' knowledge that gives power to its possessors. Reiff also (1974, p. 451) argues that the sharing of knowledge threatens the professionals' authority; therefore, the *control* of knowledge is the source of professional power.

Quint (1965) wrote a compelling article on the control by physicians and nurses of information given to women diagnosed as having breast cancer. She found that clients were often given only vague generalities about their cancer and surgical procedures, that clients were not told precisely about the extent of the cancer found during surgery, that doctors and nurses made it difficult for clients to ask direct questions, and that the impediments were even greater when the cancer was more extensive. Not only did these actions protect the professionals from having to discuss death or dying, but they prevented clients from taking control of their illness and their future life plans. Another study (Davis and von der Lippe 1967, pp. 336–344) described the negative sanctions used by physicians when clients did take control by leaving the hospital against medical advice (AMA). Lorber (1975, pp. 213–215) says that the withholding of information from clients is a way in which doctors and nurses try to minimize criticism of their work. She found that clients who asked questions and did not passively submit to professional authority were labeled "problem" clients.

The traditional balance of power between health care professionals and clients has existed for a very long time. What is happening to change it? What factors have led to the increased consciousness of health care consumers? Wolfe (1971, pp. 530–532) writes that clients now want increased control over their own health care because of the following factors: (1) a feeling that quality health care is a basic human right; (2) a higher level of education and income, leading to greater expectations for health care; (3) an increased skepticism of big government and big business and the information they provide; and (4) a desire to be more directly involved in the decisions that affect their welfare.

Much of this shift in the attitudes of consumers was due to the political and social developments of the 1960s and 1970s. People became disillusioned with the way in which the government handled the war in Vietnam and became dissatisfied with standard avenues for citizen participation such as voting and petitioning. There were mass demonstrations and protests. The civil rights movement and its associated legislation spurred on those who had felt deprived and discriminated against in the past. The inadequacies of our health care system were publicized more and more on television and radio, and in the newspapers. The increased status and power of consumers in general, led by Ralph Nader, was bound to spread to the field of health care. As a result of all these political and social developments, the public, including health care consumers, began questioning and challenging the "special" knowledge of professionals. As the social distance and level of knowledge narrowed between the consumers and providers of health care, clients began demanding more information about and the opportunity to participate in their own care.

In the light of these developments and in the hope of bringing about more effective and satisfying patient care, the House of Delegates of the American Hospital Association (AHA) approved the "Statement on a Patient's Bill of Rights" on February 6, 1972. This statement appears to have been a turning point in the awareness of clients' rights both for professionals and consumers.[1] The Bill of Rights is as follows:[2]

1   The patient has the right to considerate and respectful care.
2   The patient has the right to obtain from his physician complete current information concerning his diagnosis, treatment, and prognosis in terms the patient can be reasonably expected to understand. When it is not medically advisable to give such information to the patient, the information should be made available to an appropriate person in his behalf. He has the right to know, by name, the physician responsible for coordinating his care.
3   The patient has the right to receive from his phsyician information necessary to give informed consent prior to the start of any procedure and/or treatment.

[1]A literature search on clients' rights in the *New York Times Index* and the *Reader's Guide to Periodical Literature* revealed that most lay articles on clients' rights appeared after the AHA statement was published.

[2]Reprinted, with permission, from "A Patient's Bill of Rights," published by the American Hospital Association.

Except in emergencies, such information for informed consent should include but not necessarily be limited to the specific procedure and/or treatment, the medically significant risks involved, and the probable duration of incapacitation. Where medically significant alternatives for care or treatment exist, or when the patient requests information concerning medical alternatives, the patient has the right to such information. The patient also has the right to know the name of the person responsible for the procedures and/or treatment.

4   The patient has the right to refuse treatment to the extent permitted by law and to be informed of the medical consequences of his action.

5   The patient has the right to every consideration of his privacy concerning his own medical care program. Case discussion, consultation, examination, and treatment are confidential and should be conducted discreetly. Those not directly involved in his care must have the permission of the patient to be present.

6   The patient has the right to expect that all communications and records pertaining to his care should be treated as confidential.

7   The patient has the right to expect that within its capacity a hospital must make reasonable response to the request of a patient for services. The hospital must provide evaluation, service, and/or referral as indicated by the urgency of the case. When medically permissible, a patient may be transferred to another facility only after he has received complete information and explanation concerning the needs for and alternatives to such a transfer. The institution to which the patient is to be transferred must first have accepted the patient for transfer.

8   The patient has the right to obtain information as to any relationship of his hospital to other health care and educational institutions insofar as his care is concerned. The patient has the right to obtain information as to the existence of any professional relationships among individuals, by name, who are treating him.

9   The patient has the right to be advised if the hospital proposes to engage in or perform human experimentation affecting his care or treatment. The patient has the right to refuse to participate in such research projects.

10   The patient has the right to expect reasonable continuity of care. He has the right to know in advance what appointment times and physicians are available and where. The patient has the right to expect that the hospital will provide a mechanism whereby he is informed by his physician or a delegate of the physician of the patient's continuing health care requirements following discharge.

11   The patient has the right to examine and receive an explanation of his bill regardless of source of payment.

12   The patient has the right to know what hospital rules and regulations apply to his conduct as a patient.[3]

Most of these espoused rights for clients mean that they can participate in areas that were previously viewed as the domain of health care professionals.

[3]Despite the language of the AHA Bill of Rights (referring primarily to "doctors" and "medical care"), its relevance to *nurses* and *nursing care* is undeniable.

It appears that the most outstanding issue that has blocked client participation in health care has been the lack of knowledge. If clients are to have new rights, it would seem that health care professionals also have new obligations to see that those rights are not interfered with and are, in fact, upheld. It is the role of the advocate to see that both the client and the health care system undertake a new learning process. The client needs to learn more about his or her body, the health care it requires, and his or her rights in the health care system. The nurse-advocate needs to give up ideas of authority and control over the client, share knowledge with the client, and be a role model for other health care professionals in an attempt to change the health care system and make it more responsive to the needs of clients.

THE NURSE AS CLIENT ADVOCATE

The nursing literature has increasingly mentioned the role of the nurse as client advocate (see "References" and "Suggested Readings"). Jeanne Quint (1965), discusses the nurse's role in upholding the client's right to participate in decision making where his or her life and future are affected. This includes clarifying misconceptions and keeping the client informed about all facets of his or her care in order to prevent information discrepancies.

The National League for Nursing (1959) has had a statement of client rights for about two decades. The statement recognizes that good nursing care requires a collaboration between the consumer and the provider of care.

Kosik (1972) writes about her nursing experience in a large, urban ghetto setting. The clients were generally poor and uneducated. She exercised an advocate role in helping clients fight their way through insensitive and highly bureaucratic agencies. When she witnessed the inhumane treatment of one client, she wrote a letter documenting the situation and sent copies to five hospital and clinic directors; her letter eventually led to a resolution of the problem.

Bayer and Brandner (1977, p. 86) suggest that nurses should withdraw from the efforts of the health care system to maintain authority over health care consumers, but rather support the efforts of consumers to make their own choices. They view the nurse as a consultant to the client, sharing ideas for solutions to problems and exploring the consequences of each. Ultimately, though, the client must decide which alternative will be implemented.

In a study of health professionals' attitudes toward consumerism in health care, nurses scored significantly higher (more positive) than physicians (Van Kempen 1976). This may be a function of nursing's traditional involvement in many phases of a client's life, as opposed to medicine's primary focus on disease. The nurse is often aware of a client's moment-to-moment concerns, questions, and expectations, and is, therefore, perhaps more apt to advocate the client's rights to have such questions and needs answered. The same study showed a significantly positive correlation between professionalism and attitudes toward consumerism, indicating perhaps that nurses see advocacy as professional behavior and that professional autonomy for nurses encompasses their right to include clients in the decision-making process.

CASE EXAMPLES

The following are case examples where the nurse acted as a client advocate.

Case 1

Many hospitals are now including a copy of the Bill of Rights in the information given to clients on admission. The nurse-author went to work in a hospital where this was not the practice. A client was given the Bill of Rights only if requested. Needless to say, since most clients were not aware of the bill, very few requested it. The withholding of such information by omission perpetuates the powerless, unknowledgeable position of clients. The author resolved to find out who controlled the dissemination of this information, why it was so restricted, and whether or not a change in this policy was being considered. She learned that this issue was being dealt with not by the client care committee (which has nurse representation) but by the medical executive board (which does not). She also learned that the proposal had been ''in committee'' for months. She encountered some difficulty in trying to find out what this proposal was or who could tell her about its current status, (for example, had it been tabled or was it being actively revised or pursued?). Therefore, the author requested a position on the patient care committee in the hope of introducing a Bill of Rights proposal there.

The nurse as advocate has a responsibility to find out what the powerful committees are in an agency and to make sure that they have nurse and consumer representation. Of particular importance is nurse and consumer membership on those hospital and/or agency committees that are directly concerned with health care and client rights. This is important because nurses alone cannot guarantee clients' rights; the agency's administrators and physicians must also know about and support these efforts.

Case 2

Mrs. R. was rooming in with her 3-year-old son, Tommy, who had suffered a concussion when he fell from a grocery cart. During the hospitalization, both mother and son contracted the flu. Mrs. R. was admitted to the hospital when her asthma flared up; she was assigned to a room on the fourth floor, two stories above her son.

Mrs. R. was very concerned about how her son would feel about her absence. She thought she ought to be permitted to room in since she and her son both had the same illness. Tommy would frequently call for his mother after awakening and throughout the day. Mrs. R's parents would visit Mrs. R. and relate how much Tommy missed her. Then Mrs. R. would get upset and demand either visiting privileges or discharge so that she could begin rooming in again. On Saturday, the nursing supervisor, Ms. D., received one call after another: the grandparents felt Tommy was not recuperating because of maternal deprivation and loneliness (he was on isolation); Mrs. R. felt Tommy was not receiving good care and so she was calling the pediatric floor continually to ask the nurses to check on Tommy; the pediatric nurses did not want Mrs. R. to visit because of the possibility that she might infect the other children; the staff on the fourth floor were unable to get Mrs. R. to cooperate in her own treatment because she was so preoccupied with her son.

Ms. D. acted as a client advocate to try to clear up the tangled communications and work out a solution *with* Mrs. R. Ms. D. arranged a meeting with Mrs. R., the grandparents, Tommy, a nurse from pediatrics, a nurse from the fourth floor, and the infection control nurse. Both Mrs. R. and the grandparents aired their concerns. The infection control nurse said that it would be all right for Mrs. R. to room in with Tommy if both of them remained on respiratory isolation and wore masks whenever they left their room. The advantage of this arrangement was that Mrs. R. could assume responsibility for most of her son's care and would be there whenever he called. A disadvantage was that she would probably not get enough rest and sleep.

Another alternative was suggested by the pediatric nurse. Mrs. R. would remain on the fourth floor. Whenever Tommy awoke and called for his mother, the pediatric nurse would call to inform Mrs. R. who could then decide whether she wanted to come down to see him. Mrs. R. added that the nurses could assume responsibility for bathing and dressing Tommy, but she wanted to be able to eat her meals with her son. With this plan she would have several rest periods during the day and be able to get a good night's sleep.

Mrs. R. considered these two alternatives, as well as a third (discharge against medical advice for both her and her son) and decided on the second one. Ms. D. assured her that the nursing staff of both units and both physicians would be informed about this arrangement. The plan was successfully implemented for the four remaining days the two were hospitalized.

Acting as the client's advocate, Ms. D. had clarified a confusing, misunderstood situation. She had also made the health care system (in this case, two hospital units) responsive to the unique needs of Mrs. R. and Tommy. In the process, Ms. D. acted as a role model for the other relevant nurses, indirectly educating them about the advocacy role. Most importantly, the advantages and disadvantages of several solutions to this problem were identified and discussed with Mrs. R., and she was able to choose which solution she preferred. This intervention fits the definition of advocacy since it increased the client's autonomy and self-determination.

Bayer and Brandner (1977, pp. 86–87) call this process nurse/patient peer practice—a problem-solving approach where it is the *client* who solves the problem. The authors write about the advantage of the nurse and the client pooling their suggestions for a solution, thereby giving the client more alternatives from which to choose.

Tryon and Leonard (1965, pp. 120–126) utilized a similar approach on the matter of a predelivery enema for women in labor. When the enema was presented as a choice with the advantages and disadvantages listed, not one woman refused. These women reported that the nursing staff were significantly helpful during their stay, whereas such helpfulness was not reported by those women in the experimental group who were not given a choice about the enema.

Case 3
A third example of advocacy concerns Ms. F., a 54-year-old woman with bilateral mastectomies and extensive bone metastases. She was aware of her diagnosis and took an interest in every aspect of her treatment. She had read a great deal about her illness before her current hospitalization two weeks earlier for cobalt therapy to a newly discovered lesion in her lumbar spine. Ms. F. was very much concerned about obtaining relief for her pain. She was in continuous pain, which was being relieved only with Dilaudid 3 mg every 2 or 3 hours, intramuscularly. She was very discouraged about the pain, wondering how long she could put up with it; she hated the grogginess she felt after each injection. She was angry that nothing was being done to bring her relief and felt that in this day and age there must be other alternatives than "getting stuck with a needle all the time."

One evening she heard about Brompton's cocktail on television; it is a mixture of narcotics, antiemetics, alcohol, and flavoring and is widely used in England and Canada to relieve chronic pain. She asked her nurse, Ms. S., about the mixture. Ms. S. said she had heard of the mixture and would get more information. Ms. S. went to the library and found an article on the subject; she made three photocopies—one for Ms. F., one for herself, and one for Ms. F.'s doctor, Dr. K.

Ms. S. then made an appointment with Dr. K. She told him about Ms. F.'s frustration and her questions about Brompton's mixture. She said that Ms. F. was an intelligent, well-read individual who would like to know what other possibilities might be able to relieve her pain. Dr. K. said that since Ms. F.'s bone lesions were estrogen-dependent, a hypophysectomy or adrenalectomy could be performed, or a new experimental antiestrogen drug could be tried. He said, however, that he had decided that Ms. F. would probably not tolerate surgery well, and that he did not have much faith in the experimental drug. He was also skeptical about the use of Brompton's mixture and said he would prefer to change the narcotic. Ms. S. told Dr. K. that she believed Ms. F. should have the choice of what should be done to manage her pain. However, in order for Ms. F. to be able to make a decision, she needed to know the pros and cons of the various alternatives that were available to her. Dr. K. argued that "patients" could not make decisions of such magnitude because they could not possibly comprehend all the consequences. Ms. S. countered that it was their (the doctors' and nurses') responsibility to make sure that their clients *did* have the necessary information to make choices about their care and treatment.

After further discussion for another half hour, Dr. K. said that if Ms. S. wanted to give all this information to Ms. F., then she, the nurse, would have to be responsible if the patient's chosen treatment did not work. Ms. S. said that she would assume responsibility for seeing that Ms. F. received accurate information about the various alternatives, but that the final choice and its consequences would be Ms. F.'s responsibility. Ms. S. agreed to share the complete information about the alternatives with Dr. K. for his validation before discussing them with Ms. F. Ms. S. also assured Dr. K. that he could still make his recommendation known to Ms. F. Ms. S. took these important steps to try to make Dr. K. an ally rather than an adversary. She wisely chose to collaborate with the physician rather than put Ms. F. in the position of having to decide "whose side" (the doctor's or the nurse's) she would take. At the same time Ms. S. defended her belief in Ms. F.'s right to make her own decisions.

Ms. S. obtained information on five alternatives for Ms. F. to consider: (1) use of Brompton's mixture, (2) use of the experimental antiestrogen drug, (3) adrenalectomy, (4) hypophysectomy, and (5) use of more than one of the above. The information about each included the cost, side effects, complexity of procedure, length of treatment, length of hospital stay, length of effectiveness (pain relief), possible risks, and whether or not a cure was possible. This information was validated by Dr. K. who said that he disagreed with this approach but was curious to see what would happen.

After mulling over the information and asking several questions, Ms. F. decided on a hypophysectomy with the use of Brompton's mixture before surgery and after surgery if the pain should reappear. Even though hypophysectomy has been successful in relieving pain only 50 percent of the time, and then only for a year on the average, Ms. F. felt that the risk was worth taking. Ms. F.'s anxiety and anger were significantly reduced as she began to feel that she was once again in control of her life.

This example also illustrates the definition of advocacy: by increased knowledge, Ms. F. gained some autonomy and self-determination. Another important point is made as well: the nurse as client advocate must be willing to disagree openly with the doctor, to become highly involved with a client, and to be responsible and accountable to a client for the accuracy of the information shared. Ms. S. did not wait for the physician to tell her what to do, but took independent, responsible action based on her conviction that clients have a right to participate in the critical decisions that affect their lives.

THE FUTURE OF ADVOCACY

As discussed throughout this chapter, there are concrete ways in which every nurse can act as a client advocate. However, many aspects of health care are generally unknown to consumers, and there is little or no consumer input. These areas include the management and control of health care agencies, the performance record (infection rates, deaths in the operating room, accidents to clients, and so forth), the rate of waste, and the financial status of agencies (charges and profits). It is a shame that the only time consumers are allowed to know about or participate in any of these matters is usually when legislation requires it.

Finally, the one area that is especially "off limits" to health care consumers is their own health care records. According to the American Hospital Association, clients have a right to complete and up-to-date information about their cases in language they can understand. However, the physician still has the prerogative to decide *how* complete and *what* the client can and cannot understand. In only a handful of states are health care records available to clients without litigation (Golodetz et al. 1976, p. 78). Not all clients want to see their records; however, for those who do, a viable alternative might be the use of a single, ongoing health record that would be in the possession of the health care consumer. In this way, the client could keep informed and there could be a continuity of care since the client would carry the record to each agency that is utilized. There are also disadvantages to this method (loss of records, expense of duplication, lack of understanding of terms in record, and so forth), but it is a worthwhile approach to consider.

Another issue pertaining to client advocacy is whether or not an agency should have a separate position for patient advocate, client representative, or ombudsperson, as they are frequently called. At first glance it might seem logical to have one person who would concentrate exclusively on the task of advocacy. It also seems reasonable to assume that if each nurse was functioning as an advocate, a separate position would not be required. When discussing the creation of such a position, one needs to consider the following:

1   Will the client advocate be a nurse or not?
2   What will be the priorities of this person? Obviously, the advocate will not be able to see each and every client.
3   What will be the method for obtaining feedback from clients? Oral? Written?

4 Will the advocate take care of complaints himself or herself, or simply refer them to various other departments?

There are two major objections to having a separate office of client advocate: (1) only a small percentage of clients could be contacted, whereas, if each nurse practiced the role, all clients could conceivably benefit; and (2) a separate office would be just one more addition to an already overly fragmented health care delivery system. It would seem better to have nurses, whom the clients know, implement the advocacy role with each of their client groups.

These and other matters must be the concern of the client advocate. All nurses, as advocates, should be responsible for keeping informed about current trends and issues in health care and for lobbying on behalf of their clients' rights.

SUMMARY

Being a client advocate can be risky. It may require making unpopular decisions, having disagreements with physicians and other personnel, and commiting oneself to a very great extent in the personal lives of clients. Advocacy can also be very rewarding for the nurse because the results (for example, increased client satisfaction and control, decreased anxiety and anger) are usually highly visible. The other advantages and disadvantages that have been discussed throughout this chapter are summarized in Table 12-1.

An advocate has been defined as one who increases the client's au-

Table 12-1 Advantages and Disadvantages of the Client Advocate Role

Advantages	Disadvantages
More *client-identified* needs are met	Requires time and energy to inform clients
Client cooperation is increased because of greater control of his or her life and health	Requires flexibility in routine
Communication is improved between nurse, physician, client, and family	Requires cooperation between the nurse and physician and a breakdown of the traditional adversary relationship, which some believe is an impossibility
Responsibility for the consequences is shared with the client since he or she shares the responsibility for decision making	Requires the giving up or sharing of power or authority with the client
	Increases the conflict with other health care professionals who do not want to share their knowledge or authority

tonomy and self-determination. A word of caution: the level of autonomy desired by each client will differ. The goal of advocacy is to uphold the client's right to participate to the extent that he or she chooses in making decisions affecting his or her life and health. Nurses are in an ideal position to be client advocates; they often have the important initial contact. Every nurse has the capacity to practice advocacy to the degree that he or she is willing to admit clients into partnership to help preserve their dignity and autonomy. The nurse as advocate has a responsibility to see that both the client and health care system are educated about their new roles and responsibilities in the provision of health care.

REFERENCES

Bayer, Mary; and Brandner, Patty. 1977. Nurse/patient peer practice. *American Journal of Nursing* 77,1:86–90.

Davis, Milton S.; and von der Lippe, Robert P. 1967. Discharge from hospital against medical advice: a study of reciprocity in the doctor-patient relationship. *Social Science and Medicine* 1,9:336–344.

Dodge, Joan S. 1972. What patients should be told: patients' and nurses' beliefs. *American Journal of Nursing* 72,10:1852–1854.

Friedson, Eliot. 1974. Professions and the occupational principle. In *Professions and their prospects,* ed. Eliot Friedson. Beverly Hills, Calif.: Sage Publications, pp. 19–38.

Golodetz, Arnold; Ruess, Johanna; and Milhous, Raymond. 1976. The right to know: giving the patient his medical record. *Archives of Physical and Medical Rehabilitation* 57,2:78–81.

Kosik, Sandra Henry. 1972. Patient advocacy or fighting the system. *American Journal of Nursing* 72,4:694–698.

Lorber, Judith. 1975. Good patients and problem patients: conformity and deviance in a general hospital. *Journal of Health and Social Behavior* 16,6:213–225.

Quint, Jeanne C. 1965. Institutionalized practices of information control. *Psychiatry* 28,5:119–132.

Reiff, Robert. 1974. The control of knowledge: the power of the helping professions. *Journal of Applied Behavioral Science* 10,3:451–461.

Statement on a patient's bill of rights. 1972. Chicago: American Hospital Association.

Tryon, Phyllis; and Leonard, Robert. 1965. Giving the patient an active role. In *Social interaction and patient care,* ed. James Skipper and Robert Leonard. Philadelphia: Lippincott, pp. 120–126.

Van Kempen, Shelley Ann. 1976. *Professionalism versus consumerism: an exploratory study of health professionals' attitudes.* Master's thesis, Rutgers University.

What can a patient expect of modern nursing service? 1958. New York: National League for Nursing.

Wolfe, Samuel. 1971. Consumerism in health care. *Public Administration Review* 31,5:528–536.

SUGGESTED READINGS

Annas, George J. 1972. *The rights of hospital patients*. An American Civil Liberties Union Handbook. New York: Avon Books.

————. 1974. Rights of the terminally ill patient. *Journal of Nursing Administration* 4,2:40–44.

Bandman, Elsie; and Bandman, Bertram. 1977. There is nothing automatic about rights. *American Journal of Nursing* 77,5:67–72.

Haug, Marie R.; and Sussman, Marvin B. 1969. Professional autonomy and the revolt of the client. *Social Problems* 17,3:153–160.

Kelly, Lucie Young. 1976. The patient's right to know. *Nursing Outlook* 24,1:26–32.

Kramer, Marlene. 1972. The consumer's influence on health care. *Nursing Outlook* 20,9:574–578.

Pankratz, Loren; and Pankratz, Deanna. 1974. Nursing autonomy and patients' rights: development of a nursing attitude scale. *Journal of Health and Social Behavior* 15,9:211–216.

Vincent, Pauline. 1970. Do we want patients to conform? *Nursing Outlook* 18,1:54–55.

Community Health Agencies: An Alternative to Institutionalization

Joan Schroeder and Rita DeCotiis

OBJECTIVES

After studying this chapter, the learner will:

- Define a home health agency
- Define the management process in a home health agency
- Describe the internal and external forces that promote change in the delivery of home health services
- Explain why home health care is a viable alternative to institutionalization

Health care provided in an institution is costly to the consumer from both a monetary and human viewpoint. With the present system of health care, it is imperative that various alternatives be considered. Such alternatives must be recognized and expanded in order to be utilized effectively. One alternative that is currently underutilized is the community home health agency; it is in a position to provide services on all six levels of care as described by Clark and Shea in Chapter 1.

DEFINITION OF A HOME HEALTH AGENCY

For those who are not familiar with home health care today, a brief description of this subsystem is in order. As early as 1877, visiting nurse agencies in many areas of the country made nursing visits to the ill at home regardless of their ability to pay. Title XVIII of the Social Security Act (or Medicare), which was enacted in 1965, included home health benefits for those over 65; consequently, home health agencies have flourished.

To be eligible for Medicare reimbursement, a home health agency must meet the criteria for certification as set forth in the conditions of participation and outlined in the Federal Register. An agency must offer nursing and at least one other discipline, such as physical therapy or speech therapy. Today, the range of services offered varies—from the agency that provides only nursing and one other discipline to one that employs a variety of health professionals, such as physical therapists, occupational therapists, speech therapists, nurse practitioners, medical social workers, and home health aides. A variety of different organizations render these services: nonprofit voluntary agencies, hospital-based home care departments, official agencies (county or local health departments), and, in some areas, proprietary or profit organizations.

MANAGEMENT OF A HOME HEALTH AGENCY

The management process in a home health agency, as in any organization, utilizes human and material resources to accomplish the organization's goals. The functions of management include planning, creating, designing, coordinating, controlling, and evaluating. These components are not isolated but interdependent and dynamic. Programs and goals change, shift, and grow as do community and client needs. The nurse in management must be aware of trends and be able to assess needs. By encouraging creativity and innovation among staff members and by utilizing their skills as well as those of other knowledgeable professionals, managers can benefit in their role as leaders. Goal setting and decision making must finally rest with the manager, but employees should be encouraged to participate actively in these processes. A free flow of communication establishes an open system, which is vital to any health organization. In order for an organization to establish and implement an effective management system, it needs clear, two-way channels of communication between management and staff. There should be an ongoing evaluation of this system.

Many home health agencies have the same type of bureaucratic structures as hospitals. The problems that nurse-administrators face in this bureaucracy depend upon their positions within the system. Power and control in decision making and goal setting may be very limited because of restrictions imposed by higher levels of administration. This is most often evident in agencies with a political or hospital affiliation where the nurse functions at a middle management level.

The nurse-administrator of a voluntary, private home health agency has the benefit of less organizational rigidity. In such an agency, limitations usually arise from a lack of resources rather than from restrictions on the manager's authority or decision-making power. Under ideal circumstances a board of directors trusts and supports the nurse-manager it has hired. The manager has freedom in determining staffing patterns and needs, filling positions, and setting salaries within the budget framework worked out with the board. In fact, this is a major part of the manager's activities; other activities include interpreting community health needs to the board, to the consumers in the communities served, to physicians, and to third-party payers. In order for the agency's strategies to be effective, the manager must interact successfully with all of these groups.

Because they are more autonomous, nurse-administrators in a nonaffiliated home health agency must be highly competent in skills that are only incidentally related to the nursing profession. They must continually increase their knowledge of fiscal management, economics, business administration, health and political trends, and theories of organization and administration—to name but a few areas. At the same time, they must be aware of advances in the practice of nursing and of other health professions. They must also continue their practical experience, utilization of available human and material resources, and education. Today, professional nursing education is very limited, considering the diffusion and complexity of the modern community health system. Consequently, agencies may want to hire business managers, public relations specialists, grantsmanship experts, and others with specialized skills to help management. Although the cost would be exorbitant for a small agency, larger agencies have found these resources to be invaluable.

One trend in community-based home health agencies is to hire as chief executives nonprofessionals who have expertise in management. Professional health care direction is then provided by an assistant director of nursing, who takes charge of all the professional disciplines. With the need for increasingly complex and diverse skills to administer a health facility effectively, such specialization (with dual responsibility and authority) may be one solution for home health agencies.

It is essential to guard against the building of yet another bureaucratic health system that places the professional nurse in a strictly functional position, with little or no decision-making power or authority. However, the freeing of professional nurses from some administrative tasks could enable them to perform better in the areas of planning, creating, coordinating, and evaluating health service programs. These and the other functions of management would continue to be interdependent throughout the organization so that there would be interaction between these two facets of administration.

Community home health agencies, especially private, voluntary ones, seem to be in the best position at present to effect changes in their administration and organization because they are less subject to bureaucratic and medical components than are large institutions. These agencies—through innovative, creative, and knowledgeable administrations and boards of directors—may be able to take a new approach to the whole concept of organization and thus meet health needs more effectively. However, one of the greatest drawbacks is the lack of material resources; the administrator often spends an inordinate amount of time and energy trying to raise money.

UTILIZING INTERNAL AND EXTERNAL RESOURCES TO PROMOTE CHANGE

Change is required for any organization; without it, an organization, whether a large, profit-making business or a small home health agency, would cease to function. However, before any change can be made, there must be an assessment of need, and then planning and implementation. For example, if an analysis of statistics demonstrates that there is a rise in cardiovascular disease in a community, there is a need for screening and counseling programs to identify and educate high-risk clients as early as possible. The agency may have to use both internal and external resources to develop and implement such a program.

Internally, a free-standing voluntary home health agency has four main components that must enter into any effort to effect change: the board of directors, the executive director, the professional advisory committee, and the staff. The board of directors in this type of agency is usually composed of members of the communities served by the organization. Since this board is the ultimate policy-making body, its composition is of the utmost importance. The members should represent the various socioeconomic groups residing in the area and possess the necessary expertise for such a board; lawyers, accountants, bankers, and politicians might well serve as members. Inactive, uninformed persons on the board would constitute a great barrier to effecting change. A dynamic board is one that provides leadership, service, understanding, and commitment.

New board members need a thorough orientation to all facets of an agency's operations, including its strengths and weaknesses. Operating under agency bylaws, the board meets at regular intervals. During the 1970s most agencies have had to increase the number of meetings to keep pace with the expansion of home health services. The number and role of committees appointed by the board vary from agency to agency, but one essential committee is the advisory committee. Under federal regulations for participation in Title XVIII, the board must appoint members of the medical, nursing, and therapeutic professions, as well as consumers, to this committee. Medical advisory committees have long been well established; however, consumer participation in policy and program review is relatively new. The professional advisory committee plays a major role in the agency's operation; it reviews and advises on all policies and procedures that relate to the delivery of health services. New programs cannot be implemented until they have been reviewed by this committee. The opinion of this group is then communicated to the board of directors for final approval or disapproval. Composition of the professional advisory committee must be considered as carefully as board membership. A physician who does not perceive home care as a major subsystem of the health care system or does not understand the expanded role of nursing would be a poor choice. Knowledgeable consumers who feel comfortable about communicating objectively with professionals would make desirable committee members.

The board of directors appoints an executive director, who acts as liaison between the board and the staff. Although the management functions of the director have already been discussed, it is important to emphasize that the director must be cognizant of all internal and external forces that effect change. Figure 13-1 shows that this position carries with it the responsibility for a vast flow of communication.

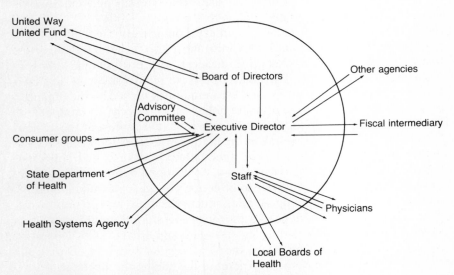

Figure 13-1 Flow of communication in a home health agency.

The staff must participate in any change process. The staff provides services not within the subsystem of the agency but in the larger system of the client and environment. Because of their highly developed skills in assessment and evaluation, the staff should be able to identify many unmet needs and provide constant feedback to the agency. If the community health nurse does not possess these skills, there are fewer chances of implementing change.

The federal government has done more to effect change in home health service than any other external force by providing money and requiring adherence to rigid regulations. The home health agency continues to feel the influence of the federal government through Medicare and Medicaid regulations, especially with each revision or reinterpretation of the conditions of participation. Federal mandates have brought about the implementation of utilization review, nursing audit, and program evaluation, for example.

Federal funding through grants also allows for the expansion of existing programs or the establishment of new ones. The astute administrator who wishes to start an innovative program to improve the health of the community will find that this source has been virtually untapped by home health systems. The authors' agencies received money through Title I of the Housing and Community Development Act of 1974 to set up health consultation walk-ins throughout the area. Monies from this act had previously been granted for physical improvements such as roads and sewers. Social and health services, not often considered visible by community leaders, did not receive priority rating. To act as agents of change, the directors of the agencies had to attend community meetings and convince the decision makers of the value of health care programs of this type.

In January 1975, Congress enacted Public Law 93-641, which mandated the establishment of Health Systems Agencies. This law and its regulations, which are discussed in Chapter 15, have had a great impact on home health care. Each local area, whether an individual county or a group of counties, has been charged with formulating a plan for the delivery of health care so that it is accessible, cost-effective, beneficial to the consumer's health, and non duplicative in services. The federal government has made a serious effort to encourage the development of alternatives to the traditional health system and to evaluate the advantages and disadvantages of the various alternatives. Home health agencies must participate actively with the Health Systems Agencies in order to be recognized in the overall health plan as a major component in the delivery of services. At the same time, they must make every attempt to assure quality and control costs.

Local government can also be utilized to maximize the home health agency's services. In many communities, local board of health nurses serve in the areas of disease prevention and health promotion, while the home health agency cares for the ill at home. Such a situation produces fragmentation in nursing services. Those with political clout in the community should be approached and informed about the advantages of a single system of nursing services. Arguments in favor of the single-system approach may vary from cost-effectiveness to the better continuity of health services. Local boards of health are financed by the municipal budget and therefore find it difficult to add staff members to meet new needs; the voluntary home health agency, on the other hand, has a much more flexible budget and several sources of income.

Bringing about a change in a community can be a cooperative venture among the existing health organizations. For example, the American Lung Association has been funding (through grants) the education and use of nurses in specialized respiratory home care programs. Similarly, the American Heart Association has helped to finance other demonstration projects in home care. Professional organizations such as the American Nurses Association, the National League for Nursing, and the American Public Health Association—with their expertise and national prominence—can help to exert pressure for change in the present health care system. Statewide organizations of agencies, such as the Home Health Agency Assembly of New Jersey, have been helping organizations improve the quality of care through communication and coordination. Such statewide organizations can urge more comprehensive health programs.

Finally, community group such as senior clubs, service associations, and church organizations can be approached not only for financial backing but also for their moral support of new programs. A local government needs the confidence of its leading groups and will listen if enough groups speak out. The power of community groups in bringing about change cannot be underestimated. Consumers—either individually or in groups—must be educated to know what to demand in the delivery of health care. Linking internal and external forces in the change process can lead to a holistic approach to health care for the single client and an entire community.

HOME HEALTH CARE AS A VIABLE ALTERNATIVE
TO INSTITUTIONALIZATION

Most home health agencies have grown rapidly and are striving continually to augment the services they offer, but they are still underutilized. In a recent three-year period, less than 1 percent of the money spent for health care was used for home visits. Institutional care has become the accepted standard for many reasons, including the relative ease with which third-party payers can reimburse an institution and the physicians' convenience in having all their clients in one place. However, the General Accounting Office reports that 25 percent of this country's client population is treated in facilities that exceed the needs of the client. As far back as 1965, the State of New York Governor's Committee on Hospital Costs recommended that hospitals be used primarily for clients whose condition could not be treated outside a hospital. Clearly, as shown by the health delivery situation today, the recommendation has not been followed.

The Council of Home Health Agencies and the Community Health Services of the National League for Nursing created a model for home health benefits consisting of basic services, other essential services, and desirable environmental-social support services. Basic services include: nursing, home health aide/homemaking, physical therapies, occupational therapies, speech therapies, nutritional counseling, social work, and medical supplies and equipment. Other essential services include: audiological, dental, laboratory, and ophthalmological services; physicians' care; podiatry; respiratory therapy; x-ray services; housekeeping; home-delivered meals; client transportation and escort; prescription drugs; and prosthetic and orthotic services. Desirable environmental-social support services include: barbers and beauticians, handymen, heavy cleaning, legal and protective services, pastoral counseling, recreational services, translation services, and personal contact (such as friendly visitors). The first group of services could be provided either directly or by contract. Some of the other services could be developed with volunteers. Obviously, if all or many of these services were available, there would have to be considerable planning and coordination by an agency. Rather than establishing a new agency, a community should add these therapeutic services to the present functions of the home health agency that is already serving the area. Available community resources such as Meals on Wheels, Friendly Visitors, FISH (a voluntary transport group), and the Red Cross should be utilized. Furthermore, outpatient facilities to which clients could be transported for dental, ophthalmological, podiatric, x-ray, and laboratory services should be examined and utilized.

Under the present-day American health care system, the physician devises the medical plan of treatment for managing each case. Federally mandated PSROs will eventually have more control over the way in which hospital services are utilized. Advocating either earlier hospital and nursing home discharge or total care at home, the authors would suggest that a physician initiate a referral to a home health agency and, together with the client and family, decide what services are needed. A plan of care could then be established. Clients would be accepted for home care if the guidelines were met; primarily, this would mean a safe and adequate home environment.

The levels of home care might be categorized as intensive, intermediate, and maintenance. Clients could be admitted to the home care system at any of these levels, depending upon their condition and needs; and they could progress from one level to another. The frequency and duration of the services would vary in intensity and would include instruction and guidance about necessary care, including information about medication and its side effects, special diets, and exercise routines. Periodic medical, nursing, and other therapeutic assessments could be planned for clients on a maintenance level (those whose conditions are stabilized but chronic). In order for the client to remain at home, additional services such as meals, transportation, housekeeping, and other chores might be necessary.

Two typical case studies will be presented, demonstrating the effective use of coordinated health care in the home. In a local community hospital during a 6-month period, twenty-one persons over age 65 were diagnosed and admitted with fractured hips. The treatment for each client included the insertion of an Austin Moore prosthesis. As a group, these clients spent a total of 407 days in the hospital, or an average of 19.4 days per person. Three persons under age 65 stayed 42 days, or an average of 14 days per person.

Case 1

The following case, though fictional, shows how the use of a coordinated home health program could reduce costs while supplying quality care during recovery. Ms. Jones, aged 60, was admitted to the hospital on January 2, 1977, after having sustained a fractured left hip. On the same date, surgery was performed and an Austin Moore prosthesis inserted. The client had an uneventful postoperative course, responding well to physical therapy. After consultation with the client and discharge coordinator, the physician determined that Ms. Jones could be discharged on the ninth postoperative day, with a referral for home care. The other alternative was for Ms. Jones to spend approximately five additional days in the hospital. Home care was chosen and the plan as shown in Table 13-1 was established.

Progress

After the first week, the client was sufficiently independent to remain at home alone during the day. The home health aide was discontinued, but intermittent physical therapy and nursing visits continued. By the end of the second week, Ms. Jones had progressed to the use of a straight cane in ambulation. Her gait was good, strength improved, and balance was excellent. The client was discharged from intensive home care to a basic program where the nurse would check back in one month to assess her condition. Arrangements were made during the second week for community meals to deliver two meals a day. This was to be continued until such time as the client was able to drive. In addition, the local Red Cross was contacted to provide transportation for Ms. Jones' visit to the physician. Table 13-2 shows a comparison of the costs between home care and hospitalization.

Table 13-1   Home Care Plan

Discipline	Frequency of visits	Plan of treatment
Physical therapy	Three times a week for 2 weeks	1 ROM exercises active and passive to both lower extremities for increased mobility and muscle strengthening 2 Gait training—walker; progression to quad cane and straight cane 3 Instruction of aide in gait training and active ROM regime
Nursing	Twice a day for 2 weeks	1 Supervise HH aide 2 Restorative nursing 3 Check incision line
Home health aide	8 hours for 5 days	1 Assist with personal care 2 Assist with ambulation and ROM exercises per physical therapist 3 Meal preparation, shopping 4 Laundry

Case 2

The following case history was taken from the records of a home health agency. Ms. B., 75 years of age, was referred by a local physician for intensive home health care when no bed was available in the local hospital. On January 12, 1977, she suffered a cerebrovascular accident with right hemiparesis and aphasia. Before this crisis, the patient had been an alert, active widow who lived alone in her own home. Her only daughter lived in a neighboring town. The plan of treatment as shown in Table 13-3 was instituted as an emergency measure until hospital space was available.

Progress

Ms. B. progressed in one week from being a client in bed with complete dependence in ADL to partial independence in self-care and transfer with

Table 13-2   Comparison of Costs

Cost of home care*		Cost of additional hospitalization†	
5 days home health aide services 8 hours per day	$180.00	5 days at $145 per day room and board	$725.00
4 nursing visits	54.00	5 physical therapy treatments at $25 per session	125.00
		Total	$850.00‡
6 physical therapy visits	96.00		
Rental of walker, quad cane	7.00		
Total	$337.00		

*Based on 1977 charges—Nursing Service, Inc., Ridgewood, N.J.
†Based on 1977 charges—a local community hospital.
‡This figure reflects only the base charges.

Table 13-3   Home Treatment Plan

Discipline	Frequency of visits	Plan of treatment
Nursing	Every day	1 Instruct aides in care of client, including positioning and skin care 2 Check intake and output 3 Restorative nursing—passive ROM and transfers; follow up on PT 4 Check vital signs 5 Assess need for equipment
Physical therapy	Three times a week	1 Bed activities—ROM exercises to all extremities and instruction of aides 2 Balancing 3 Ambulation when feasible
Speech therapy	Evaluation	1 Evaluate need for therapy and set up treatment plan
Home health aide	(24 hours per day initially)	1 Personal care of client in bed, including bathing, skin care, positioning 2 Record intake and output 3 Follow up on physical therapist's instructions 4 Keep record of medications and administer to client as dispensed by the nurse 5 Prepare meals for client 6 Keep client's room and linens clean
Occupational therapy		1 Whenever feasible if client is not hospitalized

supervision. By the end of the second week, she was ambulating with a walker under supervision and was transferring bed to chair and chair to walker independently. The night aide was discontinued and the daughter remained in the home during the period from 6:00 P.M. to 6:00 A.M. A speech therapy evaluation showed that the client was regaining verbal communication, and the therapist felt that treatment was not needed. Nursing visits recorded one elevation of blood pressure, which was reported to the doctor. With a change in medication, the client's blood pressure fell to within normal range. Occupational therapy started in the third week. The therapist worked with fine motor activities of the right hand and the activities of daily living. Visits from these disciplines were decreased as the client progressed. By March 24, 1977, the physical therapist's discharge summary stated that the client had made a remarkable recovery, regained full ROM, ambulated well with a cane, and was able to climb stairs. The client was discharged to the basic care level, to be seen by a nurse monthly for a health assessment. Table 13-4 compares the total costs of the two forms of care.

Table 13-4 Comparison of Costs*

Cost of home care†		Cost of hospital care‡	
Home health aide—14 days (2 twelve-hour shifts at $40 per shift)	$ 896.00	17.6 hospital days at $145 per day room and board	$2552.00
28 nursing visits	378.00	17 therapy visits using three modalities at $25 per session	425.00
22 physical therapy visits	352.00	1 speech therapy visit	30.00
1 speech therapy visit	18.00	4 occupational therapy visits	80.00
4 occupational therapy visits	64.00		
Rental of hospital bed	90.00		
Rental of walker	4.00		
Rental of quad cane	3.00		
Total	$1805.00§	Total	$3087.00§

*This comparison is based on the average length of a hospital stay for a CVA (17.6 days). It does not take into consideration the fact that home care usually follows a hospital stay for Medicare patients with a CVA.
†Based on 1977 charges—Nursing Service, Inc., Ridgewood, N.J.
‡Based on 1977 charges—a local community hospital.
§This figure does not include any other hospital costs.

ECONOMIC AND PSYCHOSOCIAL IMPACT

These case studies mainly analyzed the economic feasibility of rendering care to clients in their homes. The other important consideration is the psychosocial benefits to persons who can remain in their own homes after an accident or illness. This often occurs in the case of terminal illness where the client and family prefer home care to institutionalization, given adequate support systems. Instead of being socially isolated in an impersonal facility, the client is able to receive the necessary emotional support from the family. Together with professional assistance, it is possible for the family to work through the grieving process and ultimately achieve acceptance. A client can often make the transition from illness to the highest level of attainable health more quickly when he or she is in familiar surroundings. The elderly often cannot adjust to institutionalization and may regress. It has been found that many people improve more rapidly at home when they return to their usual patterns of daily living.

As mentioned previously, reimbursement by a third party is more readily available for institutionalized clients than for those receiving home care. In fact, most home health and skilled nursing benefits are tied into a prior hospitalization, which accounts for unnecessary admissions and abuses of the present health care system. However, many bills have been introduced into the U.S. Congress to remedy this situation.

In 1975, the New Jersey Medicaid regulations were revised to include coverage for intensive, intermediate, and basic levels of care in the home.

As of 1978, the State Office of Medical Assistance was formulating guidelines to determine what type of clients would benefit from intensive 24-hour care at home rather than in an institution. New Jersey Blue Cross is examining the utilization of intensive home care and, with the cooperation of home health agencies, may develop a pilot project to assess the feasibility and cost factors. Since 1976 there has been a marked increase in the partial insurance benefits for home health care. Both New York and New Jersey have passed legislation mandating private insurance companies to include home health charges as part of the reimbursable benefits of their hospitalization policies. Thus, it appears that there may be more funding for home care.

SUMMARY

Reevaluating inappropriate and costly care in an institution and comparing it with home-centered care will have an enormous economic impact on health care in this country. Today, there are still many obstacles to home care that need to be overcome. Governmental influence and control over building, expansion, and duplication through the Health Systems Agencies (HSA) will prevent the kind of random spending that went on for thirty years. Innovative approaches and uses for present facilities will be needed, and there should be more ambulatory care centers to which clients can be transported. Services such as podiatry, dental care, vision and hearing testing, mental health, and social services could be made more accessible. Group settings for teaching and other therapeutic regimes could be encouraged. In general, hospitals ought to reach out to the community at large and share their facilities and expertise (in both treatment and prevention).

It is essential to have built-in methods for evaluating expanded home care programs for quality and effectiveness. These might include utilization reviews, professional units, uniform cost accounting and cost containment systems, outcome statistics, and consumer feedback.

To compete with the greater visibility of such towering buildings as a medical center and to sell society on the advantages of clients remaining at home whenever possible during illness or disability, home health agencies need to face critical social and health care issues. New public policies and innovative long-range health planning must be considered. Consumers of health care must be made aware of this alternative, perhaps to the point where they think of institutionalization as their *second* choice. Perhaps treating clients for specific needs in their own environment will the the basic form of health care in the future.

REFERENCES

Council of Home Health Agencies and Community Health Services. 1974. *Proposed model for the delivery of home health service*. New York: National League for Nursing.

Freeman, Ruth. 1970. *Community health nursing practice*. Philadelphia: Saunders.

Graves, Helen Hope. 1971. Can nursing shed bureaucracy? *American Journal of Nursing*. 71, 3:491–494.

Hamil, Evelyn M. 1969. The changing director of nurses. *Nursing Outlook*. 17, 12:64–65.

Health is a community affair. 1966. *Report of the National Commission on Community Health Services*. Cambridge, Mass.: Harvard University Press.

Home Health News and Review. 1975. National Association of Home Health Agencies, December.

Inquiry. 1967. Volume IV, No. 2. Blue Cross Association, October.

Simon, Herbert A. 1957. *Administrative behavior*. New York: Free Press.

———. 1965. *The expanding role of the ambulatory service in hospitals and health departments*. New York: New York Academy of Medicine.

———. 1975. *The techniques of nursing management*. Wakefield, Mass.: Contemporary.

U.S. Department of Health, Education and Welfare. 1973. *Home health in China-town*. Washington, D.C.: U.S. Govt. Printing Office.

Chapter 14

Political Methods

Marian Martin Pettengill

OBJECTIVES

After studying this chapter, the learner will:

- Define the political process
- Define power base
- Define the legislative process
- Identify the factors that influence the political activism of nurses

DEFINITION OF THE POLITICAL PROCESS

The political process offers nurses one means for instituting change. To understand the political process, nurses need to know: (1) What is politics as it pertains to nursing practice? (2) What is a power base? (3) What is the legislative process? and (4) What factors influence the nurse's use of the political process to institute change? For this discussion, politics is defined as the art or science of government that shapes and influences public policy (Novello 1976, p. 1; Bowman 1973, p. 73). Individuals within the political system use the system to effect change by assuming that their goals and ideals require governmental sanction and funding. The legislative process, one aspect of government, provides an arena in which the individual or group can influence the governmental system. Although Mullane states that the political process begins with one's own institution or agency since politics is necessary for any social group or enterprise to function (1975, p. 699), only the political process as it relates to government will be considered here.

DEFINITION OF POWER BASE

Basically, the political process involves influence, and power is the source of influence (Claus and Bailey 1977, p. 21). The greater the power, or the ability to act in relation to others, the greater the political persuasion that can be exerted to control those who hold similar goals or ideals. Power requires an interpersonal reference point that is covertly or overtly understood; power is generally derived from any of five sources (Novello 1976, p. 3):

1   The ability to punish or coerce.
2   The ability to reward.
3   The ability to know, which comes from knowledge, skill, and expertise.
4   The ability to exercise influence through the allocation of resources—both people and things.
5   The ability to exercise referent power which arises from people's expectations of a certain role.

Thus, power is potentially available, at any given time, to those who are willing to expend the energy and resources required to influence others (Morgenthau 1967, p. 157). Since power exists on an interpersonal level, the more one seeks it, the more one becomes its potential master and subject.

Power exists in five forms: (1) exploitative—power *forced upon* persons for the use they may have to the one who holds the power; (2) manipulative—power *over* another person, which may be initiated by that person's own desperation or anxiety; (3) competitive—power *against* another, which may be either negative or constructive in nature; (4) nutrient—power *for* the other; this is seen in the normal parents' care for their children and in statesmanship; and (5) integrative—power *with* the other person, which *abets* another's power (May 1972, pp. 105–110). All five are found in an individual and system at different times; the crucial questions are, however: In what proportion? At what time? and in what place?

Power, in whatever form, gives access to a situation. Access is strengthened by the status and prestige of the power-seeker(s) and by the resources—either monetary or informational—offered by the power-seeker(s). Nurses can enhance their power with legislators by applying the concept of reframing, which means:

> To change the conceptual and/or emotional setting or viewpoint in relation-ship to which a situation is experienced and to place it in another frame which fits the "facts" of the same concrete situation equally well or even better, and thereby changes its entire meaning. . . . What is altered is the meaning attributed to a situation and, therefore, its consequences, but not the con-crete facts (Watzlawick, Weakland, and Fisch 1974, p. 95).

The practical use of reframing for political action is seen in the various positions taken on the New York State Nurses Association's proposed 1985 resolution that espouses the baccalaureate degree for entry into pro-fessional practice. The facts—the need to upgrade the profession and to reduce fragmentation within nursing education and service—remain the same; however, one group of nurses view these facts as threatening to their existence, whereas another group uses these facts to try to ensure the future of nursing. Nurses try to influence other nurses as well as legis-lators by altering the meaning of these facts to try to obtain what they believe is in the best interests of the profession. As one group of nurses tries to exert influence on the legislative process, another group is trying to restabilize the system. Each legislator interfaces with other legislators, his or her constituents, and the nurses seeking change, and tries to assess the information received. The amount of power exerted by all forces within the system, the readiness of the system to realign its steady state, and the openness or closedness of the system all help to determine the amount of disequilibrium that will be tolerated before there is a return to a steady state.

Power can either cause or prevent change (May 1972, p. 99). Change in the political process means either the enactment or amendment of legis-lation or the establishment of statutory regulations and guidelines for in-terested groups or individuals. Today individuals have little power, and so they form groups to exert political pressure. "An interest group becomes a political pressure group when it attempts to influence governmental de-cisions, either directly or indirectly, without placing its members in formal governmental capacities" (Bowman 1973, p. 74). Political action, then, is a secondary interest of the group. An interest group is seen as a collection of individuals who, "on the basis of one or more shared attitudes, makes certain claims upon another group in the society for the establishment, maintenance, or enhancement of forms of behavior that are implied in the shared attitudes" (Zeigler 1966, p. 30). The strength of a pressure group depends upon the degree of its formalization and cohesiveness, the extent of its personal resources and alliances, the size of its membership, and the amount of its monetary wealth. The pressure group's effectiveness varies according to society's needs and priorities at any given moment, and with the popularity of the issue under consideration. Hence, timing is extremely important; it can either make or break the effectiveness of a pressure group in trying to influence a policy-making group.

Through lobbying (providing technical and political information), political pressure groups intervene in the policy-making process of government (Bowman 1973, p. 78). The accuracy and reliability of the information is vital because it (1) informs legislators of significant public attitudes, (2) provides research data and speech material, and (3) gives credence to the trade-off of mutual support. Nurses are active lobbyists, although it is not clear whether the lobbyist for a nurses association should or should not be a nurse. A nonnurse lobbyist who is skillful in the political arena may help to break down the stereotype of the nurse, whereas a nurse lobbyist can directly confront the issues and convey an independent and authoritative image.

The power utilized by political pressure groups does not exist within a vacuum; it is a dynamic force, charged by the interplay of human relations which are at the core of the political process. While the legislative process provides the arena, how individuals use it to play the power game with others is of the utmost importance. One must vigilantly observe and evaluate the environment and the other players in the power game (Bowman and Culpepper 1974, p. 1056).

THE LEGISLATIVE PROCESS

One must understand the legislative process in order to be effective in playing and winning the political power game. The mechanics of the political process are relatively simple and are the same whether approached by an individual or a group. A goal or ideal is stated and governmental sanction is sought. The individual or group then meets formally or informally with an appropriate legislator or member of the executive branch. If agreement is reached on the need for such legislation, a bill is written and sponsor(s) are sought in the hope of securing legislative approval. The proposed legislation may remain a very long time in committee, where legislators argue the merits and pitfalls of bringing the bill to the floor of their legislative branch. Once a bill does reach the floor, it may be voted upon, tabled, or sent back to the committee for further study. If the bill is passed, further approval is needed by the other legislative branch before executive action is taken.

Obviously, most of the work on impending legislation takes place in committee and is completed before presentation to the other members of the legislature. The procedural differences among the states and the federal government, though slight, need to be reviewed separately in order to understand the specific nuances (Nathanson 1975, p. 1179).

Figure 14-1 shows the legislative process in New York State; it was prepared by the New York State Nurses Association to assist nurses in understanding and making use of the legislative process. As can be seen in the figure, there are certain important points of access where one must assess the strengths and weaknesses of the assemblymen and senators, provide pertinent information, and demonstrate widespread support. One also needs to know who controls which committee, what form of power is most appropriate, which district the legislator represents, when he or she will be up for election, the current fiscal stresses within the system, and what power is being exerted by allied and conflicting groups in the health field. After a bill has been enacted, the pressure groups that supported it must monitor its implementation by providing information for procedural guidelines and regulations and in other ways ensuring that its intent is carried out.

Three valuable resources—local elected officials, the League of Women Voters, and the political action arms of state nurses associations and the American Nurses Association—can provide nurses with information so that they can understand the local, county, state, and federal governmental systems. It is ironical that the political process, which requires the use of power to influence, should all too often be imbued with magical powers that intimidate nurses from participating in it.

NURSES IN THE POLITICAL PROCESS

It is striking that while nurses were the first health profession to support the concept of national health insurance, nurses have actually just begun to take an active role in trying to influence governmental policy making. The political activity of nurses in the past and present has somewhat paralleled that of the women's movement. This is not too surprising since nurses have been predominately women, with a slow and small influx of men into the profession in recent years. What is more significant is that the women's movement today far surpasses that of the nursing profession as a pressure group with an influential power base.

Forces that Influence Political Activism

Nurses ought to analyze why they have been hesitant to utilize the political process as a vehicle for change. Why women have not been as suc-

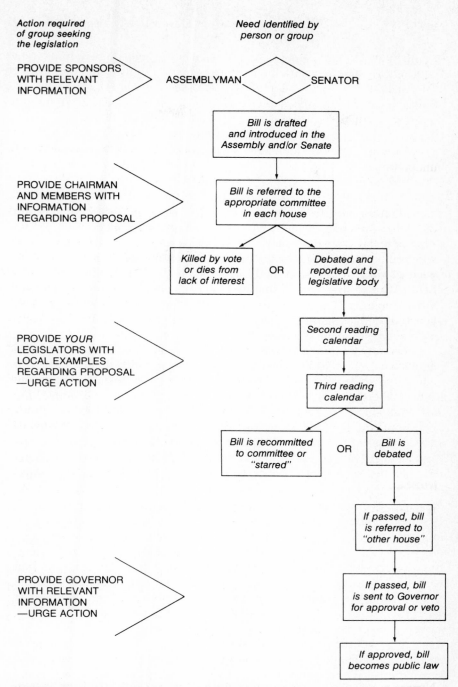

Action required of group seeking the legislation

PROVIDE SPONSORS WITH RELEVANT INFORMATION

PROVIDE CHAIRMAN AND MEMBERS WITH INFORMATION REGARDING PROPOSAL

PROVIDE *YOUR* LEGISLATORS WITH LOCAL EXAMPLES REGARDING PROPOSAL —URGE ACTION

PROVIDE GOVERNOR WITH RELEVANT INFORMATION —URGE ACTION

Need identified by person or group

ASSEMBLYMAN   SENATOR

Bill is drafted and introduced in the Assembly and/or Senate

Bill is referred to the appropriate committee in each house

Killed by vote or dies from lack of interest   OR   *Debated and reported out to legislative body*

Second reading calendar

Third reading calendar

Bill is recommitted to committee or "starred"   OR   *Bill is debated*

If passed, bill is referred to "other house"

If passed, bill is sent to Governor for approval or veto

If approved, bill becomes public law

Figure 14-1 The legislative process in New York State. (Reprinted with permission of the New York State Nurses Association.)

cessful as men in the political process can be attributed (but not limited) to
the following factors:

1   Feelings of and actual demonstrations of powerlessness (Bowman
and Culpepper 1974, p. 1054).
2   Actual and assumed naïveté and innocence.
3   Dependency on and submission to male authority (in institutions
and agencies).
4   Alienation of self and the profession.

These factors help to put nurses in a defensive, nonassertive position
where they are predominately passive. Passivity limits one's effectiveness
in the political system on such vital issues as revised practice acts, third-
party reimbursement, inclusion on PSROs, professional entry into practice, and nurse traineeship funds. Unless nurses take an active role, few
changes can be made on these issues. Because nurses can achieve power
by participating in a group and by identifying with the power of their
agency of employment, they have not demonstrated personal power outside the employment situation (Cleland 1971, p. 1542).

This may be due to *feeling* powerless as individuals, or that powerlessness and submission are part of the nursing socialization process. If it
is assumed that nurses *are* powerless, they may be defeated within the
legislative process or within their own organizations. For example, the
American Nurses Association has established a policy on certification for
practitioners at baseline levels and for certain divisions of practice at advanced level of practice. At various times pressure groups such as the
Council of Advanced Practitioners, the New York State Nurses Association, and the Society of Certified Clinical Specialists in Psychiatric Nursing of the New Jersey State Nurses Association have tried to alter and
expand the American Nurses Association's requirements for Advanced
Psychiatric Mental Health Certification. As each group has worked to
influence the ANA, it has experienced helplessness and powerlessness;
obviously, an integrative effort is needed to challenge a large system.
Eventually, such activities as active letter writing, personal confrontation
with the appropriate ANA committees, phone conversations with the
ANA's leaders and publicity of the issues to nurses across the country
were utilized to deal with this issue of certification; finally, the ANA
agreed to hear the opinions of the interested parties and to discuss the
issue. Whether the American Nurses Association will alter its standing on
advanced certification requires constant attention by the concerned pressure groups. Without monitoring, there will be a return to the original
equilibrium, the system will close, and the subsystem groups will experience powerlessness.

Nurses' powerlessness, as perceived by others and assumed by nurses, is nurtured by innocence and naïveté (Goren 1976, p. 26). Many nurses feel that the political process is either too intricate or a masculine function. Until recently, this naïveté was common among women in general and among nurses in particular. Much of this innocence can be viewed as a defense to deny the existence of the inherent power of nurses and to ward off their involvement in the interpersonal game of politics. For nurses to participate in the political process means that they must take risks and utilize inputs in order to receive positive feedback. Assertive, not aggressive, behavior has led society to view nurses more positively, and nurses have been rewarded with certain legislative sanctions for professional practice. Revised nurse practice acts that promote and protect professional practice have been implemented in many states. Obviously, to achieve such changes means that nurses had to overcome their powerlessness and actively utilize their power.

Failure to achieve power perpetuates the myth of powerlessness; it may be attributed to either unrealistic or inappropriate goals, or the failure of the chosen intervention to reframe the facts of a situation (Watzlawick, Weakland, and Fisch 1974, p. 113). Nurses should stop being timid in their requests, and try to evaluate and analyze thoroughly what they want to change. The timing of the planned access into the political process must be appropriate; the language must be understandable to the agents of change; and the issues presented must be relevant to the system at that given moment. The legislation on mandatory continuing education for nurses illustrates these points. The present emphasis on peer review and updating clinical practice indicates that continuing education is a vital issue to the health care system, the nursing profession, and individuals within each system. In some states where nurses have urged mandatory continuing education legislation, it has passed and is being implemented. In other states, individual nurses have challenged the need for mandatory continuing education by providing legislators with different information, which has resulted in negative feedback and maintenance of the status quo. In still other states, mandatory continuing education is just not a top priority concern of their legislatures or regulatory bodies. In these states nurses could: (1) propose omnibus continuing education legislation to the other health professions; (2) continue to seek sponsorship on continuing education legislation while identifying and countering any opposing forces; (3) begin a massive education-information program with legislators and influential lay constituents; or (4) wait until another year when the system may allow easier access.

For nurses to be successful as a pressure group, they must form a united front so that the information they provide will be factual and valued. Division and dissension among nurses enables other pressure groups to gain access to the legislative system in order to work for the rejection or modification of proposed nursing legislation. Dissident groups point to the dissention among nurses in order to help preserve a steady state. Because of their numbers, nurses could be a powerful group; however, too many viewpoints can lead to capitulation and compromise with respect to goals, ideals, and professionalism. One of the major difficulties in trying to achieve passage of a professional entry into practice law is to reach a compromise and united position among the subsystems of nursing. Professional entry into practice legislation requires confronting such interest groups as Licensed Practical Nurses, diploma and associate degree graduates, and educational and nursing service systems in order to determine which ones are open to change and which ones do not want change. While the nursing subsystems work out their viewpoints, legislators receive input from lay groups and health consumers, and give output as to the climate for legislative change. In order to enact a professional entry into practice law, the existing system(s) (nursing, the legislature, and health care) must be receptive to change. Such a change requires compromise by the various nursing subsystems, and then the resulting cohesiveness and united objective must be conveyed to legislators through informational campaigns, personal contacts, presentations at legislative hearings, and coalitions with other health disciplines.

If nurses can cosponsor or endorse legislation with other legitimate health disciplines or *not* oppose legislation advocated by these other disciplines, they can seek support from these groups for their own proposed nursing legislation. Obviously, for an omnibus continuing education bill, such mutual support is required. In other instances such as the inclusion of nurses in exemption clauses (for example, in licensing legislation for psychologists), there must be a tradeoff and understanding among the professions. The competitive and exploitative power among the professions should give way to the larger need to utilize nutrient and integrative power to influence the legislative system.

For nurses to achieve a collaborative relationship with other disciplines (political pressure groups), they must give up their dependent-submissive characteristics. Such "female" traits often reveal themselves in work with male counterparts and in male-dominated professions. Given the fact that the majority of legislators are male, nurses must combat the image and perceptions that these legislators probably have of nurses and women. The male dominance of politics means that nurses must influence a male authority to institute the changes they seek. Another factor in the male-dominated political process is the social status of each legislator as it affects his or her perceptions of nurses (Lamb 1973, pp. 334–336). As nurses become vocal in politics or seek political office, they may be labeled "aggressive" or "castrating." These terms demean, intimidate, and aim to suppress the invasion of nurses into a traditionally male-dominated territory. However, the mere existence of such labels acknowledges that nurses are an influential group that must be dealt with by the system. Nurses need to use the power attributed to them by these accusations in order to move forward.

Another factor to consider is the alienation of nurses. Since the inception of health care, women as healers and then as nurses were viewed with skepticism and antagonism (Roberts and Group 1973, pp. 314–315). It was established early that males would dominate and control health care, and that women would be in auxiliary, subservient roles. Over time, this attitude became a social norm, and the auxiliary group became alienated. Nurses are alienated when they do not receive third-party reimbursement, do not secure high-level administrative health care positions, and do not influence client health care needs. When nurses are perceived as having none of the primary rights of health care providers, they become alienated from their identity as nurses and see themselves as alienated individuals. According to Ronald Laing: "Alienation as our present destiny is achieved only by outrageous violence perpetrated by human beings on human beings" (1967, p. XV). Exclusion from third-party reimbursement, from house-staff privileges, from patient care committees, from state and national health legislative committees, from hearings on professional conduct—these are all forms of violence that must be dealt with and prevented.

An analysis of legislation on third-party reimbursement for nurses establishes the need for strong communication among nurses at both state and national levels. Nurses must reconcile a basic difference of opinion within the profession—whether all nurses or only those at advanced levels of education and experience should receive third-party reimbursement. Once a compromise has been reached, there can be active lobbying. In some states, other health disciplines receive reimbursement and nurses are incidentally included; in other states, nurses are specifically excluded. The New York State Nurses Association has actively sought third-party reimbursement since 1974. Nurses have utilized their numerical power, sought access to committee hearings, made formal complaints about exclusion and harassment at hearings, initiated extensive and intensive personal letter-writing campaigns, and vigorously employed such pressure groups as Nurses for Political Action and women's groups. These actions finally led to the overwhelming passage of legislation regarding third-party reimbursement for all nurses by the New York State Assembly, despite strenuous oppositon from numerous pressure groups. During the 1977 legislative session, the bill reached the State Senate Committee on Insurance and was reported to the floor of the Senate; however, on the next to last night of the session the bill was "starred," implying that there was an insoluble difficulty. Consequently, no vote was taken and the bill died. Although the final outcome was negative, nurses had clearly exercised a lot of influence to get the bill that far along in the legislative process. Nurses in New York undoubtedly gained a lot of wisdom about the maneuvers and idiosyncrasies of the political system that will be useful in eliminating nurses' exclusion from their rights as health care providers.

Another factor that fosters alienation among nurses is that society does not identify them as belonging to a "doctorate" profession. Consequently, nurses do not have the ascribed status and power that are inherent in the doctorate. Legislators consider the doctorate as the expert in health care legislation. For example, legislation in New York State to repeal the exemption clause of the Nurse Practice Act (allowing certain individuals in state and federal facilities to give medication) has met with repeated opposition. The male-dominated Department of Mental Health has been able to bring about the defeat of this legislation. If nursing were a "doctorate" profession and had the ascribed power, such a defeat would be less likely!

The political activism of nurses has been encouraged by the establishment of a national group, Nurses Coalition for Action in Politics (NCAP), and a state group, New York State Nurses for Political Action (NYSNPA). These political action arms of formal organizations promote improved health care by encouraging nurses to become politically active in governmental affairs, by educating nurses about the political and legislative process, by helping nurses organize political action groups, by raising money for these activities to support political candidates who favor nursing issues. Since the American Nurses Association and state nursing associations cannot make political contributions, these two newly formed, unincorporated groups are a valuable source of influence. The Nurses Coalition for Action in Politics, the New York State Nurses for Political Action, and other state political action groups are independent of one another and reflect state and national concerns. For example, NYSNPA received seed money from the state association for operating costs, but not for political contributions. The bylaws of NYSNPA specify that it must separate its operating budget from its contributions, and that it must have separate bylaws, officers, and budget from that of the parent association.

The national group helps nurses who want to form political groups by providing organization information, booklets and pamphlets on the legislative process, and information on the voting records of federal legislators. In turn, state political action arms inform nurses about specific state issues, voting records of state and local legislators, and how to organize local groups to get the support of elected officials. Thus, the New York State Nurses for Political Action endorses candidates, makes campaign contributions, and offers organized volunteer power to a candidate; while individual members take such action as encouraging relatives and friends to register and vote; contacting precinct caucuses; becoming delegates to local, county, and state conventions; and running for political office. The NYSNPA has, during its short life, made nurses aware of the need for political activism.

SUMMARY

Nurses can help to effect change by utilizing the political process. To be successful in the political arena, one must know the players in the game, use certain strategies and appropriate timing, and have sound information on the issues. For too long nurses have been dependent on individual nurses to implement change; now, action by pressure groups is required. When power is used to confront the legislative system, the actors in the system—legislators, regulatory bodies, and consumers—must then acknowledge the position of nurses. In essence, nurses can become a dynamic force if they use their knowledge of power and the legislative process to institute change. By understanding what forces inhibit their activity, nurses can turn these liabilities into assets and then add them to their other assets as a political action group.

REFERENCES

Bowman, Rosemary. 1973. The nursing organization as a political pressure group. *Nursing Forum* 12, 1:72–81.

Bowman, Rosemary; and Culpepper, Rebecca C. 1974. Power: Rx for change. *American Journal of Nursing* 74, 6:1053–1056.

Claus, Karen; and Bailey, June. 1977. *Power and influence in health care: a new approach to leadership.* St. Louis: Mosby.

Cleland, Virginia. 1971. Sex discrimination: nursing's most pervasive problem. *American Journal of Nursing* 71, 8:1542–1547.

Goren, Sue. 1976. Innocence as an impediment to power. In *People • power • politics for health care.* Publication No. 52–1647. New York: National League for Nursing, pp. 25–32.

Laing, Ronald D. 1967. *The politics of experience.* New York: Random House.

Lamb, Karen Thompson. 1973. Freedom for our sisters, freedom for ourselves. *Nursing Forum* 12, 4:328–352.

May, Rollo. 1972. *Power and innocence.* New York: Norton.

Morgenthau, H. J. 1967. *Politics among nations,* 4th ed. New York: Knopf.

Mullane, Mary Kelly. 1975. Nursing care and the political arena. *Nursing Outlook* 23, 11:699–701.

Nathanson, Iric. 1975. Getting a bill through congress. *American Journal of Nursing* 75, 7:1179–1181.

Novello, Dorothy. 1976. People, power and politics for health care. *In People • power • politics for health care*. Publication No. 52–1647. New York: National League for Nursing, pp. 1–7.

Roberts, Joan; and Group, Thetis M. 1973. The women's movement and nursing. *Nursing Forum* 12, 3:303–322.

Watzlawick, Paul; Weakland, John; and Fisch, Richard. 1974. *Change: principles of problem formation and problem resolution*. New York: Norton.

Zeigler, Herman. 1966. *Interest groups in American society*. Englewood Cliffs, N.J.: Prentice-Hall.

Chapter 15

The Nurse as a Colleague in a Health Systems Agency

Virginia O'Halloran

OBJECTIVES

After studying this chapter, the learner will:

- Define a Health Systems Agency (HSA)
- Identify the advantages and disadvantages of this system
- Describe the role of a nurse in an HSA

DEFINITION OF A HEALTH SYSTEMS AGENCY

A Health Systems Agency is a local, federally funded health planning and regulating system. This system of health care emerged after years of unsuccessful efforts by the federal government to regulate the direction of health care in the United States. Under this system the development and regulation of health care services rests with an integrated system of local and state agencies. This system is unique in the history of federal regulation of health care in our country (Rubel 1976, p. 3). It could dramatically change the direction and quality of health care. As members of the health professions, as major providers of health care services, and as members of an HSA, nurses have a unique opportunity to influence the direction of these changes.

The National Health Planning and Resources Development Act of 1974 (Public Law 93-641) is an amendment to the Public Health Service Act. It became effective in January 1975 and authorizes the creation of a network of local Health Systems Agencies (HSAs). Each HSA develops an individualized health plan for its designated health service area and implements that plan by developing facilities, services, and manpower (*Federal Register* 1975, p. 48802).

Historical Background

The federal government has been regulating health care for many years. Its authority to do so is found in the Constitution's provision that it may "promote the general welfare" (Wilner 1973, p. 25). Over the years the federal government has been playing a greater role in health care through the establishment of various programs and the provision of funds. The National Health Planning and Resources Development Act replaces three previous legislative acts on the planning and direction of health services. Assembled into one law are the more strategic and most successful portions of the Hill-Burton Act, the Regional Medical Program Act, and the Comprehensive Health Planning Act.

The Hill-Burton Act, enacted in 1946 and amended through the years, is best known for its provisions for financing the construction and modernization of hospital facilities. Through this act, the federal government fostered other health related activities. It required states to identify their health needs and to develop plans to meet these needs on a statewide level. States were encouraged to use federally designed guidelines and standards for evaluating their facilities. Finally, in 1964, an amendment to the act created local planning councils for health facilities (*Trends affecting the U.S. health care system* 1976, p. 91).

The Regional Medical Program Act, enacted in 1965, was the next most influential piece of federal legislation. It provided grants to medical schools, hospitals, and research institutions for the development of regional programs in research and education. These programs made available to others new knowledge about the diagnosis and treatment of heart diseases, cancer, and stroke. This act developed further the concept of regional planning and cooperation among health care organizations.

Then came the Comprehensive Health Planning and Public Health Service Amendment of 1966. It provided funds for the creation of state and areawide planning councils. These councils brought together consumers of health care and representatives from state and local agencies concerned with health care for the purpose of health planning (*Trends* 1976, p. 96).

Federal monies for the continued operation of the Regional Medical Program and the Comprehensive Health Planning Agencies were insufficient. Various health care providers assisted at the local level to maintain these federally created councils by providing the money or other needed services. Thus, these groups could influence decisions about health planning and the creation of health care services (*Trends* 1976, p. 97). The strongest feature of both these programs was the consumer participation. They could share in the decision making with the health care providers and the representatives of government. The experiences gained by those who participated in creating and carrying through the Regional Medical Program and Comprehensive Health Planning agency units were seen as important to the creation of the HSAs. The influence that health care providers and government officials could have in the success of the new HSAs was recognized. The law establishing the HSA provided for an eighteen-month period of transition. During that time the functions of the Regional Medical Program and Comprehensive Health Planning agencies would be gradually assumed by the newly formed HSAs. But more importantly, these agencies had the opportunity to restructure themselves and apply for designation as an HSA for their region (Rubel 1976, p. 5).

The National Health Planning and Resources Development Act establishes three levels of operation within the system. The National Council on Health Planning and Development is at the federal level and highest in the hierarchical structure. The National Council has the ultimate authority and all of its decisions are final. There are two bodies at the state level—the State Health Planning and Development Agency and the State Health Coordinating Council, which serves in an advisory capacity to the state agency. The Health Systems Agency (HSA) is the local and basic unit for the entire system. Each level functions simultaneously as an integrated unit. It is accountable to and communicates with the other levels on common areas of responsibilities (Figure 15-1).

Local Level

The Health Systems Agency can be a nonprofit, private corporation; a public regional planning body; or a unit of local government. The health service area for each HSA is determined by geography, population base, and the existence of at least one facility that can provide highly complex services (P.L. 93-641, sec. 1511). The governor of each state with the approval of the Secretary of Health, Education and Welfare, designates the regional health service areas for that state. A state may be small enough to have only one health service area, while another may have eight or more such areas. Each health service area forms its own Health

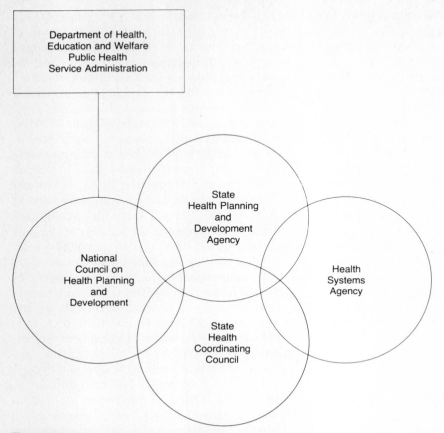

Figure 15-1   National, state, and local levels of the national Health Planning and Resources Development Act of 1974.

Systems Agency (HSA). The population of the area is normally from 500,000 to 3,000,000, but exceptions may be permitted within specified guidelines. The designated limits ensure a sufficiently large population base for effective health planning while keeping the area small enough to assure community participation at a local level (Peterson 1976, p.11). All HSA board members must be residents of the health service area and represent specific groups. Consumers comprise 51 to 60 percent of the membership and reflect the ethnic and socioeconomic makeup of the area residents. One-third of the members are direct providers of care (physicians, dentists, nurses, and other health professionals); representatives of health care insurers, health professional schools, and health care institutions; and persons from various related health professions. The remaining members represent public offices and government officials.

The major purpose of the HSA is to improve the health of those who live in a given health service area while holding down the cost of providing such health services. These services must be accessible and acceptable to the population and provide quality and continuity of care. To fulfill its purposes, the HSA carries out the following functions (*Trends* 1976, p. 105):

1 Assembles and analyzes data on the status of the health care system and that of the residents in the health service area.

2 Develops a Health Systems Plan (HSP) for the area that is in accord with the national guidelines and state plan. It considers typical health needs and services, the needs that are unique to the area of service, manpower needs, and environmental and occupational factors that affect health.

3 Develops an Annual Implementation Plan (AIP) with objectives for achieving the goals of the Health Systems Plan, establishes priorities among the objectives and provides for annual reviews and progress reports.

4 Reviews periodically all existing institutional health services in its area and makes recommendations to the state agency about their appropriateness to its Health Systems Plan and Annual Implementation Plan.

5 Reviews and makes recommendations on all proposals for expenditures of certain federal funds by private, state, or local facilities, and determines whether they are congruent with the Health Systems Plan.

6 Provides grants to public and nonprofit private groups for projects to achieve the goals of the Health Systems Plan and the Annual Implementation Plan.

7 Provides technical assistance to individuals and to public and private groups for projects that will achieve the objectives of the Health Systems Plans.

8 Coordinates its information and activities, and enters into agreements with the Professional Standards Review Organization (PSRO) in its service area as well as any other general or specialized regional planning and administrative agency.

All activities and functions of the HSA should reflect the goals and objectives of the Health Systems Plan and the Annual Implementation Plan. All of the operations are carried out simultaneously and affect one another since the activities, decisions, and recommendations of the agency bear upon each area of responsibility (see Figure 15-2). The HSA may create subarea advisory councils to assist in carrying out its responsibilities. These advisory councils follow the same federal guidelines in all aspects of their composition and function. They are represented on the HSA boards and differ only in that their recommendations are advisory in nature. Each level of the system establishes a channel of communication with the adjacent hierarchical level. The HSA exchanges information and

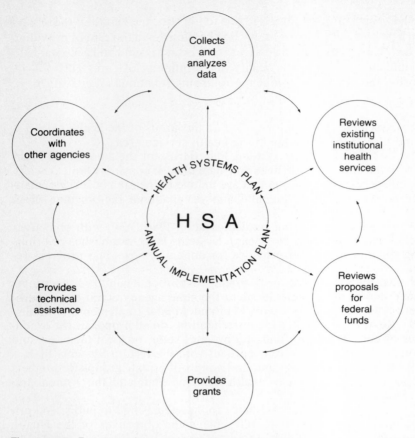

Figure 15-2 Functions of a regional health systems agency

makes recommendations to both the State Health Planning and Development Agency and the State Health Coordinating Council.

State Level

As mentioned earlier, there are two bodies at the state level. The first, the State Health Planning and Development Agency, has the following functions:

1 Prepares and implements a state health plan, which is made up of the Health Systems Plans from each HSA. This plan is submitted to the State Health Coordinating Council for review and recommendations.

2 Assists the State Health Coordinating Council in the performance of its duties and in reviewing the State Medical Facilities Plan under Title XVI of the National Health Planning and Resources Development Act.

3 Administers the certificate of need law by making final decisions on proposals for new facilities and services.

4 Reviews periodically all existing institutional health services for their appropriateness to the state's Health Systems Plans and publishes its findings and recommendations.

The second body, the State Health Coordinating Council, serves as a review and advisory council to both the state agency and the local HSAs. Each HSA has equal representation on the council. An HSA has at least two representatives on the council, one of whom must be a consumer of health care. The council is also made up of providers of care and representatives of government agencies. The governor may appoint persons whom he or she feels would be appropriate members of the council. The council has the following functions:

1 Reviews and revises the HSAs' Health Systems Plans and Annual Implementation Plans.

2 Assists the state agency in preparing, reviewing, and revising its State Health Plan.

3 Reviews the annual budget for each HSA, reporting its comments to the Secretary of Health, Education and Welfare.

4 Reviews and makes recommendations on all applications for federal funds under specified legislation.

Both the state agency and the state council communicate with the National Council on Health Planning and Development at the federal level. If an HSA wants funds, its proposals or requests are sent to the national council, the state agency, and the state council. The national council will not act on an application until it has received and studied the review and recommendations from the state level and the appropriate regional HSA. Public hearings are required at various stages of the review process in order to permit reactions and opinions from the residents in the health service area. The proposal or project is reviewed for its appropriateness to the health plans of the state agency and the local HSA. If the proposal is to initiate or expand a health service (and there is no request for federal funds), then the national council does not see it; the review process is otherwise the same, but the final decision is made by the state agency. The state agency reports annually to the national council on its State Health Plan, indicating what changes have been made in the state's facilities and services since the last report.

Federal Level

The National Council on Health Planning and Development is located within the Public Health Services Adminstration of the Department of

Health, Education and Welfare (Rubel 1976, p. 4). This council advises the Secretary of Health, Education and Welfare on the drawing up of national guidelines that are consistent with the national health priorities established by Congress in P.L. 93-641. It reviews and makes decisions on requests for federal funds, taking into consideration the recommendations made by the regional HSA, the state agency, and the state council. The national council is responsible for assisting with the implementation and administration of the HSA law.

ADVANTAGES AND DISADVANTAGES

The National Health Planning and Resources Development Act is comprehensive and future-oriented. It has the capability of assuring that greater numbers of persons receive quality health care at a reasonable cost. The strengths of the law are obvious, but there is also the potential for manipulation, mismanagement, and inequity. Nurses, as knowledgeable health professionals and members of HSAs, can help in many ways to preserve the intent of the law.

Each HSA covers a specific geographical area and provides a complete range of health services to individuals and families who live within the area. Thus, those who live in the outer regions of a state can receive the same quality of health care as the residents of metropolitan areas. The law facilitates the regionalization of health care services—the concentration of complex health services in one large facility within a health service area. Careful monitoring is needed to make sure that specialized services remain within the local community facility despite regional trends. An HSA can intervene, if necessary, to preserve a community-based service. The following case illustrates this point.

Case History
As the birth rate declined in one particular area, the need for a maternity unit in each of the two community hospitals was questioned since it was rather costly for the institutions. One hospital was located at the western end of the county and the other at the eastern end. The state health department began to press for the closing of maternity units in hospitals across the state, but especially in metropolitan or suburban areas. Hospitals that did not meet specified occupancy levels or delivery rates per year were strongly urged to begin planning to centralize maternity services in one larger hospital facility. However, the closing of the one particular maternity unit would have created a serious hardship and would have been against the health and welfare interests of the residents of that area. If that maternity unit were closed, some of the area residents might have to drive for more than thirty minutes over back roads to reach another maternity facility. The regional HSA helped to set up a series of meetings with hospital representatives, physicians, and the

state health department. After lengthy discussions the HSA sent a letter supporting the continuation of both hospitals' maternity units. The state health department temporarily ceased its efforts to close the hospital unit.

The initiative taken by the HSA in this case demonstrated that mutual cooperation among hospital, physician, state, and consumer representatives can effectively resolve a community problem. The regional HSA was influential in making recommendations to another government agency.

The National Health Planning and Resources Development Act provides federal funds for the total estimated operational needs of the system at each level. More money is allotted for the HSAs under this act than had been allotted for programs under previous health legislation. Furthermore, health care providers cannot receive funds or other services under this law. Thus, the health care provider is less likely to try to influence the actions of the HSA board members. Financial indebtedness is one form of manipulation; however, board members need to be cognizant of less obvious forms of manipulation. All proposals must receive critical evaluation and appropriate recommendations. HSA members must be free of outside influences when making decisions. Nurses should try to enlighten consumers and others about potentially manipulative situations that are cached in well-meaning health programs.

The composition of the HSA board is carefully outlined in the law; although a mixture of various ethnic and socioeconomic groups is mandated, this does not guarantee that the less aggressive economically deprived consumer will find a place on the HSA. The methods for nomination and appointment to the HSA board need to be widely publicized. All subgroups of a community need an opportunity to be represented and to help make health care decisions for their area. Since nurses and their colleagues know the community and its leaders, they can help to facilitate the nomination and election of these individuals to the HSA board. There would be less opportunity for politically wise individuals to be consistently reappointed to the HSA if other qualified individuals were readily available.

The HSA must write a Health Systems Plan for its area and spell out step by step how the plan will be implemented for the ensuing year. Each level of the system is monitored by means of written reports and public hearings. Unfortunately, neither the state agency nor the HSA have the power to *require* changes cited as necessary; the federal or state government regulates changes through legislation, while the HSA or state agency attempts to influence others to change. Public notices alert community groups and encourage them to take action in effecting such changes. Government agencies, which are put on notice, can regulate the necessary changes. Decisions and recommendations made by the HSA are essentially advisory in nature. It is not clear whether the HSA can realistically influence or reverse decisions made at the state or national level on controversial issues. An alert, informed, and involved community is the best monitoring system. Nurses should try to encourage community participation on particular issues and alert consumers to the implications of health proposals for them as clients.

The HSA coordinates its activities with all other appropriate general or specialized regional planning or administrative agencies in its area (P.L. 93-641, sec. 1513). Communication among the groups within the system is mandated and formalized. This helps to reduce the duplication in data gathering, increase cooperation among different parts of the health care system, and facilitate implementation of the Health Systems Plan. Monitoring is needed to make sure that the close cooperation among health care groups does not lead to supporting special interest projects that benefit only a minority of the residents in the area.

The HSA helps to administer the certificate of need program, thereby being in a better position to effect changes in its area, lessen duplication efforts, and reduce costs. The certificate of need law prevents the creation of unnecessary health facilities and services by requiring that a need for them has been established. Since consumers comprise a majority of the HSA members, they have an opportunity to make decisions that will add or change facilities or services in their area. However, consumers need clear and accurate information on the scope and impact of a proposed service (Pecarchik 1976, p. 75); this is a responsibility of the health professionals and others on the HSA.

An important provision of the National Health Planning and Resources Development Act is the establishment of a uniform cost accounting system for all health care facilities and services. The law requires that differences in cost for health services be based on clearly defined criteria and reflect the true cost of providing services to each category of client. Such financial accountability could serve as the basis for rate regulation by state or federal agencies under a future national health insurance plan (*Trends* 1976, p. 108). The full impact of this aspect of the law needs further exploration.

The HSA is still in its infancy. It needs support, guidance, and supervision to assure that the intent of the law is fully carried out. All activities and written materials of the HSA are open and available to the public. The scheduled meetings of all regional HSAs, subarea councils, and standing committees of the region are published in the media and distributed through the mail. Agendas are available upon request and in advance of the meetings. Table 15-1 shows a sample agenda of a regular HSA meeting. Every meeting of the HSA or its committees is open, and there is a public participation period before every regular meeting. At that time, one

Table 15-1   Sample Agenda of a Regional Health Systems Agency

Maple Valley Health Systems Agency

Agenda

Date: September 27, 1977
Place: HSA office, Maple Valley, New York
Time: 4:00 P.M.

1 Public participation

2 Roll call

3 Minutes of August 23, 1977 meeting

4 Committee reports
  a Project review
  b Plan development
  c Mental health
  d Emergency medical services
  e Membership and nominations

5 Chairperson's report

6 Old business
  a Statewide Health Coordinating Council
  b Tristate Regional Planning Commission
  c Regional proposal on obstetrical units

7 New business

8 Adjournment

can bring up issues of concern or reactions to HSA services or programs. Although the usual time allotted to such matters is fifteen minutes, issues of major concern can be placed on the regular agenda of a future meeting. Furthermore, special meetings or public forums may be called to allow persons or agencies to present various sides of an issue.

The standing committees of each HSA deal with the activities that relate to its delegated responsibilities. Although the members of these standing committees must be HSA members, other ad hoc committees might have as members those who have relevant special knowledge or expertise.

THE ROLE OF THE NURSE IN AN HSA

Nurses are among the major health care providers today, and their ability to effect change is beginning to be realized. Nurses, together with physicians and dentists, are recognized as appropriate members of Health Systems Agencies. Nurses have a responsibility to seek out HSAs in their region and take an active role in these health care systems by attending meetings and serving as members of selected working committees. Each HSA has committees that correlate with areas of health need and help develop the Health System Plan. Nurses should be represented on these committees and should communicate and consult with consumers and with other nurses, health professionals, and providers of health care. These committees need knowledgeable professionals with holistic, health-oriented viewpoints. Nurses have an educational background that is health- rather than illness-oriented, and they perceive the health care needs of the whole person. They know the roles, functions, and goals of each discipline in the health care field, and they are used to articulating nursing care with an interdisciplinary team every day. Nurses focus more and more on the client's rapid return home and on assisting with development of community and family support systems. They understand the needs of the client in the community as well as in the hospital. As colleagues in HSAs, they can educate other professionals, government agencies, and consumers on the role of nursing in the health care delivery system.

Through the years, nurses have been consumer advocates; now they can help the consumer understand how the health care system functions. Consumers need pertinent data that will help them make informed decisions on health issues. They need to learn how to effect changes within health care systems. The nurse in an HSA can assist the consumer in becoming more knowledgeable and aware. Cost-effectiveness and regionalization will be offered as reasons for future changes in health care service. Nurses can help to focus attention on the unique needs of each individual and family within the system. They can alert the consumer and other professionals to the right of the consumer to be cared for within the family and community even if it is more costly.

The following are examples of how professional nurses can participate in and make decisions about health planning as well as cooperate with their fellow nurses and other professionals.

In order for a certain HSA to develop its Health System Plan, it needed to set up task force committees for each major area of health care including acute care, mental health, and home health care. Each task force in turn was responsible for developing its own Health System Plan. As the committee for home health care collected data, analyzed needs, and assessed resources, it needed a clearer understanding of the role and scope of nursing practice within that area. One nurse on the committee presented a film and spoke about the activities of nurses in a home health care agency and within the community. After this presentation, the committee members found it easier to discuss home health care and to make decisions on what levels of care should be provided for clients in this area of the Health System Plan.

Only a small number of nurses can actually serve as committee members or as members of a regional or subarea council HSA. Therefore, it is extremely important for nurses who are HSA members to represent the entire profession. As items related to the nursing profession, to nursing care, and to health care in general are brought up, nurses on HSAs must consult with other nurses in the community. This will enhance the HSA nurse member's ability to make decisions and to present various nursing viewpoints. It might be wise for the HSA nurse to establish a communication network among professional nursing colleagues. These nurses could meet at intervals, offer their opinions on materials being developed, act as consultants in nursing, and serve as a support system for the HSA nurse member who is their representative.

In one county, the HSA nurse member on the home health care committee met with nursing colleagues in the community health nursing field. They formulated broad goals for their area as it related to home care; these were then brought before the entire committee for discussion and possible inclusion within the total Health System Plan for that region. A nurse member from another county met with the directors of home health care agencies in the community. These nurse-directors reviewed and reacted to a draft proposal of the home health care section of the Health System Plan. Their suggestions were presented to the committee and to those staff members who were going to revise the draft.

As the HSA nurse member becomes more knowledgeable and experienced, he or she must assume responsibility for speaking about the HSA to professional organizations and consumer groups. The nurse can motivate others to see the HSA as a vehicle for change within the health care system. A group of informed nurses and consumers must be developed in the community so that they can be available and prepared to serve when vacancies occur on the regional or subarea council HSAs as well as on special task force committees. There ought to be a professional nurse member on every regional HSA, every subarea advisory council (where it exists), and on every working committee of the HSA.

SUMMARY

A Health Systems Agency is a local, federally funded health planning and regulating system. The National Health Planning and Resources Development Act of 1974 established three levels in the system—the National Council on Health Planning and Development under the Department of Health, Education and Welfare; the State Health Planning and Development Agency and its advisory body, the State Health Coordinating Council; and the Health Systems Agency (HSA), which is the local and basic unit of the structure. Each level of the system is an integrated functioning unit. It is accountable to and communicates with the other levels on common areas of responsibility. The purpose of the HSA is to improve the quality of health care for people in a given geographic area at a reasonable cost. The HSA is responsible for developing and implementing a Health Systems Plan for its area.

Nurses are major health care providers and as members of HSAs have an important role in determining the scope and direction of the health care system. They have a responsibility to seek out HSAs and to participate actively as colleagues with consumers, other professionals, and government representatives. Nurses bring a health orientation and holistic point of view to the health care system. They are knowledgeable professionals who can educate their colleagues as to the role and scope of nursing practice, and can bring a unique perspective to health care planning.

REFERENCES

Bicknell, William J. 1976. Critical experiences in organizing and administering a state certificate of need program. *Public Health Reports* 91,1:29–45.

Chopoorian, T.; and Craig, M. 1976. PL 93-641 nursing and health care delivery. *American Journal of Nursing* 76,12:1988–1991.

93rd Congress. 1975. National Health Planning and Resources Development Act of 1974 (Public Law 93-641). Washington, D.C.: U.S. Govt. Printing Office.

Novello, Dorothy Jean. 1976. The National Health Planning and Resources Development Act. *Nursing Outlook* 24,6:354–358.

Pecarchik, Robert; Ricci, Edmund; and Nelson, Bardin. 1976. Potential contributions of consumers to an integrated health care system. *Public Health Reports* 91,1:72–76.

Peterson, Roland L. 1976. The designation of health service areas. *Public Health Reports* 91,1:9–18.

Rubel, Eugene J. 1976. Implementing the National Health Planning and Resources Development Act of 1974. *Public Health Reports* 91,1:3–8.

Trends affecting the U.S. health care system. 1976. Department of Health, Education and Welfare Publication No. HRA 76-14503.

U.S. Department of Health, Education and Welfare. 1975. Health systems agencies: proposed rulemaking. *Federal Register* 40 (October 17):202.

Wilner, Daniel M.; Walkley, Rosabelle Price; and Goerke, Lenor S. 1973. *Introduction to public health,* 6th ed. New York: Macmillian, pp. 25–29.

Chapter 16

Action Research: For Nurses, with Nurses

Carole A. Shea

OBJECTIVES

After studying this chapter, the learner will:

- Define action research
- Compare and contrast action research with basic and applied research
- Identify six characteristics of action research
- Describe the five phases of the action-research process
- Cite two examples of how action research can be used in nursing

DEFINITION OF RESEARCH

Research is the systematic collection and analysis of data to illuminate, describe, or explain new facts and relationships (Treece and Treece 1973, p. 3). Research is a problem-solving process that utilizes the scientific method of discovery and develops ideas and theories that give meaningful answers to complex questions about humans and their environment.

There are two types of research: basic and applied. Basic research (sometimes referred to as "pure") is knowledge for knowledge's sake. This type of research is oriented toward describing, explaining, or resolving a theoretical problem by studying the effects of variables on each other as they are controlled and manipulated by the researchers. Applied research is oriented toward solving practical problems that originate in work or the social environment by applying knowledge produced by basic science or by using the scientific method (Andreoli and Thompson 1977, p. 33).

RESEARCH AND NURSING

All scientific disciplines—including nursing—rely on the research process, which combines theory and method, to guide their professional development and practice. Nursing emerged as a profession as it began to use theoretical knowledge derived from the research of basic and applied science. However, the science of nursing is more than a synthesis of knowledge from other disciplines. Rogers states that the goal of the science of nursing is "to provide a body of abstract knowledge growing out of scientific research and logical analysis and capable of being translated into nursing practice" (1970, p. 86). What is currently unique to nursing is the way scientific research is transformed into informed nursing practice.

Research in nursing is essential to provide a scientific knowledge base from which nursing theories can emerge and develop. Nursing research focuses on human life processes and supports the probability that nurses can intervene effectively to maximize the health of individual, family and social systems (Andreoli and Thompson 1977, pp. 35–36). However, the roles and functions of a nurse who deals with "the behavior of individuals and groups in potentially stressful situations relative to health and illness" (King 1976, p. 51) defy simple, abstract measurement and analysis. The complexity of nursing situations suggests that research should be carried out within a systems framework, rather than within a cause-and-effect context, to account for the interactions and interrelationships of many variables at several hierarchical levels in the health care system.

Another aspect of the significance of nursing research is the impact that it has on the health needs of clients and the delivery of health care. Research in nursing practice, that is, "client care research" relate to the management of pain, hospitalization, stress, and anxiety has led to changes in the delivery of care. Five categories of practice-related research have been identified: building the science of practice, refining the art of practice (focusing on health outcomes), establishing structures for optimal care, developing methodologies and measurement tools, and applying research findings (Gortner, Bloch and Phillips 1976, p. 23). Of these categories, the least research has been done on the application of findings. This speaks to the serious lack of implementation of nursing research, which inhibits the growth of professional nursing and tends to decrease the significance and relevance of nursing research.

Many nurse-researchers realize that accountability does not end with the writing (and publishing) of the final research report. However, due to inadequate knowledge or inexperience with planned change, nurses may not be able to proceed to the next step—the application of research findings. Also, health care organizations do not facilitate implementation when research studies are not understood, or seem out of context with organizational needs, or are likely to produce conflict because of resistance to change (Cunningham 1976, p. 215). Breu and Dracup describe the nursing administrator who must contend with the nursing staff's excuses and rationalizations when it comes to utilizing research findings. The staff may claim that the research does not apply to their particular setting; that there is no time for research because of short-staffing; or that the medical staff show no commitment or interest, or that they are suspicious and uncooperative. These researchers concluded that the utilization of nursing research requires a change in all systems, but that people naturally resist such changes in their efforts to maintain equilibrium. Therefore, in order for research to be used successfully in clinical settings, resistance to change must be anticipated and planned for (Breu and Dracup 1976, p. 14).

One method of research—action research—seeks to bridge the gap between scientific significance and social relevance, between the generation of theory and its utilization in practice. The action-research approach emphasizes collaborative problem-solving and implementation through planned change.

ACTION RESEARCH

Definition

The term "action research" was coined by Kurt Lewin, who wanted to get the researcher out of the laboratory and into "real life" settings (Lazarsfeld and Reitz 1975, p. 7). Others translated Lewin's definition of action research as the use of research methods to solve problems that are *identified by the clients* in the actual work or social system. In its broadest sense, action research is a collaborative process for achieving social change in the organizations of a complex society (Shea 1976, p. 32). Since the client is located within an organizational system, the researchers must understand and use appropriate organization and management theory in working with the client to carry out the research and implement the findings (Glaser and Taylor 1973, p. 146).

Characteristics

Action research is characterized by:

1 Direct involvement of the researcher with the research group, usually as a participant-observer.
2 Problem identification by members of the organization who are to initiate action or are obligated to respond to the action.
3 Definition of goals that are flexible, significantly important, specific, attainable, and justifiable.
4 Active participation of organization members in all phases of the research and the action.
5 Analysis of the group dynamics and environmental forces as they affect group action.
6 Implementation of results through planned change.

Action research is similar to operations research (see Chapter 4) in that both methods attempt to provide particular solutions to practical problems in organizations. Action research differs in that the action researcher introduces and observes a planned change while exploring solutions to the problem (Foster 1972, p. 534). *How* the research results are utilized is the essence of action research. Action research helps to answer the question: "Did a particular action improve conditions or change a difficult situation as anticipated?" (Cunningham 1976, p. 238).

Components

The components of an action-research project are the client system, the change agent (researcher), and the methods or approaches used to effect change. Client systems vary in such respects as size, characteristics, motivation, and so forth. The initial contact of the researchers and the research group may be made with those at the highest level of management, or with a group of persons at a lower level who perceive a need for change in the organization. Eventually, when a contract for action research has been established, the whole organization may be viewed as the client system. The change agent is a social scientist, usually an outside consultant, whose underlying commitment is to the advancement of scientific knowledge "by joint collaboration within a mutually acceptable ethical framework" (Rapoport 1970, p. 499). The change agent takes the role of researcher, consultant, teacher, trainer, and counselor, depending upon the goal to be achieved. Interpersonal skills are required, as well as technical proficiency and knowledge of research methods. Which methods will be employed depend upon the target of change—person(s), the interpersonal characteristics of groups, or the structure and its environment. In general, if form determines function, then a change in interpersonal relationships or personal insight will *not* have a major impact on organizational behavior (Foster 1972, p. 540). However, modern researchers, aware of the properties of open systems, realize that they must consider both structure and people as interacting subsystems when they plan research interventions. Interventions and the methods of research are determined by the nature of the problem and the shared philosophy and goals of the client system and the change agent.

ACTION RESEARCH AND NURSING

The action-research process is easily correlated with the nursing process. Both employ the scientific method: (1) observation (problem identification and assessment), (2) hypothesis formation (planning with rationale), (3) testing (execution of planned change and intervention), and (4) analysis and evaluation (feedback, evaluation, and revision). Action research and the nursing process are not finite activities but a series of actions that occur in consecutive cycles. Specific problems and actions change, but there is always a need for improvement or a higher level of functioning. Both processes seek the active participation of the client, recognizing the validity of the client's perceptions and the importance of the client's value system. The aim of the action researcher and the nurse is to develop competence within the client system to carry on autonomously. If action research were superimposed on the nursing process, new information about the effects of nursing interventions on the health status of clients could be collected, organized, and utilized to upgrade nursing practice while also contributing to other sciences.

Research that has real utility for consumers will be valued for itself and will bring credit to those who do the research. In the study that follows, it was anticipated that using the action-research process (rather than traditional research methods) would increase the utilization of the research findings, and enhance the esteem of the nurses who carried it out.

AN ACTION-RESEARCH PROJECT

To demonstrate the action-research process, a research study abstract is presented, followed by an anecdotal account of how the author-researcher proceeded through the first three phases of the study. For information on the utilization of the findings, see Chapter 17.

Abstract

ACTION RESEARCH WITH NURSES IN A COMMUNITY MENTAL HEALTH CENTER: A DESCRIPTIVE STUDY

The Problem Area. This study describes the process of investigating social change in a community mental health center (CMHC) using action-research methodology with a group of nurses. The participant approach of action research was used to involve those who were to take action in the research project from the beginning. Five phases were identified in the research process: (1) initiation, (2) identifying the problem, (3) problem-solving, (4) utilization, and (5) evaluation. Examples were taken from the work of the researcher with the nurses of a nursing services committee (NSC) to illustrate the development of the research project through the first three phases, with projections made for the last two phases. Indications, limitations, the control of variables, and data collection were discussed in terms of using the participant approach in a modified field study.

Review of the Literature. The literature defined action research as a collaborative process for achieving social change in the organizations of a complex society. Four areas were covered in the review: (1) the field of action research, (2) social change, (3) collaboration, and (4) organizational psychology.

Methodology. A questionnaire was devised jointly by the researcher and the nursing committee to help the nurses to study themselves with a view toward planning their future direction. The researcher used a procedure that involved the nurses as the "respondent group." The self-administered questionnaire, which covered the identified problem areas —the nurse's role, satisfactions relating to her work, and the nursing services committee's structure and function—was given to the thirty-seven registered nurses emloyed in the various units throughout the center. There were twenty-nine respondents.

Analysis, Findings, and Interpretations. The results of the questionnaire indicated that job satisfaction and morale were higher than had been anticipated. As measured in this study, clinical position, years of nursing experience, and years of psychiatric nursing experience were not significantly related to job satisfaction or morale. It was also found that the majority of the respondents wanted a director of nursing, especially those who indicated that they had no role model at the center. The overwhelming majority of nurses thought that the nursing services committee should be participating "all the time" in various administrative functions, thereby giving the committee a clear mandate to increase its level of functioning in the organization.

Conclusions and Recommendations for Further Research. Although the research study was completed before the social action could be implemented, the results of the project imply that action research is a viable method for giving clients responsibility for solving their own problems within an organizational setting. Some difficulties encountered in this nursing research project, namely, the lack of systematic planning, unilateral decision making, and the lack of time, indicate areas for further research. There is a need to develop specific programs to teach the collaborative mode of interaction to researchers and others. To increase the utilization of findings, research studies that stop short of linking knowledge and practice could be reexamined and converted into action-research projects. The findings of the questionnaire suggest that this study could be replicated in a similar CMHC with a director of nursing to determine the effects of a different organizational structure on the nurses' role. This study could also be continued through the utilization and evaluation phases with the NSC, and expanded to include a study of interprofessional relationships and problems in a multidisciplinary setting.

Phases of the Research Process

Phase I: Initiation   Action research begins when the researcher and the client first come together to begin a relationship. This often occurs through personal contacts such as mutual acquaintances, previous clients, professional conferences, or direct meeting. In this study, a faculty adviser who was also serving on the nursing services committee (NSC) put the researcher in touch with the NSC chairperson.

Right from the start there is a mutual testing-out of who needs what and who is willing to give what. Both parties need to find a genuine basis for helping each other. At this point a researcher may encounter a special difficulty in doing action research, namely, confusion about what this type of research has to offer. This stems from ambiguity in both the researcher's and other people's minds as to the role of an action researcher. This is particularly true when the researcher is new to the field of action research or has less experience with research methods in general. Those who are somewhat familiar with basic research may be startled by the researcher's proposal that they participate directly in a study about themselves. The following are typical examples of client resistance (Argyris 1970, pp. 229–230):

That's all very interesting, but we're working under great pressure right now, and we don't have time for research.

What's in it for us?

The research may upset the system.

Researchers aren't practical; they can't solve our problems.

In dealing with this resistance, which is natural and should be expected, the researcher tries to convey that he or she wants to help, and that the best way to do so is to establish a relationship with the client. Although the researcher cannot become a part of the client system and may not think as the client does, the researcher can show concern and demonstrate his or her value by thinking differently and assessing the given problem in new terms. In the beginning every effort should be made to form a collaborative relationship. The researcher must present an authentic self and avoid introducing any false note that could later produce an insuperable resistance.

In this study the researcher initiated the relationship by telephoning the chairperson, who then arranged for the researcher to attend the next meeting of the NSC to discuss her research proposal. At this first group meeting the researcher was a silent observer because urgent business did not permit time for adequate discussion of the research project. The committee was a small group that sought to establish functional norms. Stogdill's concept that "forming-storming" precedes eventual "norming" (Hirschowitz 1974, p. 233) characterized the NSC at this particular time. The members expressed their own preferred definitions of structure, process, and content. At this particular meeting when no one person would accept the nomination for chairperson, the conflict was creatively solved by electing two persons to share leadership responsibilities. In the process the members openly expressed and questioned their personal ideologies and professional objectives, as well as issues related to the organizational system. The researcher did not participate in the discussion, but was privileged to be able to remain throughout the meeting. The lively demonstration of the interpersonal and decision-making dynamics of the NSC gave the researcher an invaluable opportunity to witness the client in action. This introduction revealed such problem areas as the hierarchical structure of the CMHC, power and authority lines, nursing in relation to the other disciplines, and the nurses' performance. However, no one theme could be singled out.

The researcher was formally introduced to the research group one month later, when eight members of the NSC were attending the meeting. The researcher, who was a graduate student in psychiatric nursing, told the group about herself and her background, and attempted to describe the proposed research approach. She emphasized the importance of providing and receiving feedback about the research project, including the persons to whom she would report the information generated by this study.

Both the NSC and certain faculty of the Department of Psychiatric Nursing (who were to serve as advisers to the student-researcher) would be involved in the research process. This was an issue for the NSC, who expressed concern that there might be a conflict of interest between the two groups, the practitioners and the educators. Recognizing their suspicions, the researcher tried to assure confidentiality by agreeing to be discreet about matters relating to the sensitive areas of overlapping interest between the NSC and the Graduate School of Nursing. However, the researcher stressed the necessity of open communication between herself and the committee members in order to establish the trust required for action research. She tried to invite comments and confrontation without coercing it. As a result, she had to reiterate her position and her view of what action research is many times. Because action research is often outside the mental set of those who are more familar with traditional research, the researcher should have anticipated the need for redundancy to make sure that all members "got the message." Reclarification, careful checking out, and repeated summaries might have facilitated the development of a "public language" on action research. Another way to reach the client is to mention the questions or issues that the researcher might explore in a particular situation. These should relate to the human problems the clients may have, and the research should have a strong probability of producing insights that will lead to action (Argyris 1970, p. 233).

The initiation phase is completed when both the researcher and the client agree to continue the relationship in order to explore the possibilities for a collaborative problem-solving approach. They should both try to establish a trusting climate and to develop an understanding of the research process. That the research project is only at a preliminary stage is reflected in that there is no binding agreement to continue the program to completion. The atmosphere is one of "let's see what happens."

Phase II: Identifying the Problem During the second phase of the action-research process, both the researcher and the client try to decide what to study. It is wise to make certain assumptions about the client system (Argyris 1970, pp. 220–221):

1 Clients may have difficulty owning up to the real problem.
2 Clients may view their problems as bad or a sign of failure, and therefore the problems may cause pain.
3 Clients will generate strong constructive intentions and feel responsible for the effectiveness of the system.
4 Clients will generate strong pressures to solve the problem quickly.

5 During the early meetings, clients may unite against a preliminary diagnosis because of prevailing group forces.

Because of the likelihood of these factors, the researcher should try to draw out and clarify the client's perception of the problem. Through observation and participation, the researcher will undoubtedly have his or her own ideas as to the best focus of the study. However, clients need to conceptualize their problem in terms of their own concrete situation. Therefore, the researcher should not formulate hypotheses for presentation to the client; a premature interpretation can lead to a premature decision. He or she should facilitate questioning, searching, scanning, information-gathering, and hypothesis-generating by the group.

It was agreed that the researcher would come to another meeting to define with the NSC a problem they wanted to study, but this process actually required several meetings. The chairpersons of the committee asked the members to come to the meetings prepared to discuss problem areas in nursing. The nurses responded by talking about general matters instead of such specifics as organizational structure and power, the role of the nurse, and the need for leadership. Certain important questions emerged in relation to the construction of a questionnaire. At times, the discussion seemed like a "gripe session" rather than a step-by-step exploration of the boundaries and units of a problem and its components. Some of this digression was necessary in order to promote group cohesion. The researcher observed leadership styles and patterns of interaction that highlighted some of the problems that seemed to be inherent in the NSC. For example, the nurse clinicians dominated the meeting in number as well as in controlling communication.

At this point there seemed to be different perceptions of the problem. The researcher tried to emphasize intergroup considerations, raising the issue of collaboration with members of other professions as an area of study. The NSC was preoccupied with intragroup functioning, wanting to look at roles, objectives, and goals for nurses—especially those in the NSC. The committee could not clearly define a problem for study (or possibly the researcher could not "hear" its statement). However, eventually the problem emerged as a manifestation of the ambiguous nature of the NSC and the role of the nurse at the CMHC. The NSC rejected the researcher's suggestion of the need for better collaboration with those in other disciplines and decided to "get their own house in order" first. Toward this end, the NSC chose the following areas:

1 Comparison of the NSC's structure, function, and effectiveness with other NSCs in specific CMHCs, with and without a director of nursing.

2 Delineation of nursing service problems to help the NSC formulate and recommend potential solutions.

3 Definition of long- and short-term goals on the establishment and implementation of specific policies and procedures appropriate to effective NSC functioning.

With the NSC's definition of their problem areas, Phase II ended with an agreement to pursue research that would provide some answers. There was more commitment in the researcher-client relationship, although a formal contract had not yet been made. The researcher agreed to help the NSC undertake research on their problem, and the NSC agreed to participate actively in the process.

Phase III: Problem-Solving This phase pertains to what is done once the problem has been identified. There may be some regrouping as those who have helped to identify the problem give way to those who are pragmatic action planners. Problem-solving tasks include:

> . . . brainstorming, opinioning, the seeking of options and alternatives, the weighting and listing of these, the analysis of probable costs and consequences attached to each, and the construction of a decision scale by which to weigh alternatives (Hirschowitz 1974, p. 235).

There may be a need for more information-gathering, assessment of resources, and assignment of certain people to specific tasks. In action research, the solution should be tailored to the given problem, with the consensus of the research group.

In this study, the nurses decided—by means of extensive discussion and reports from a fact-finding mission to other CMHCs—that the NSC wanted a needs-assessment study to determine their problems and define their goals. The researcher proposed that all who were interested within the CMHC come together for the special purpose of devising a questionnaire to delineate pertinent issues and problem areas as perceived by members of all disciplines. She saw this as a means to foster collaboration at the CMHC and provide feedback to the NSC vis-à-vis their position and function within the organization.

The researcher's suggestion was indirectly rejected. The research study was labeled "C. Shea's Project." The committee members refused to recruit "interested others" themselves and insisted that the researcher do so herself. There was a general lack of enthusiasm for the whole idea, but the members voiced only vague misgivings.

The researcher persisted in considering the possibilities of her approach. However, she finally realized that she was attempting to force a solution based on *her* perception of the problem rather than the client's. This was a direct violation of the action-research principle that clients must define their own problem. The collaborative relationship was severely tested by this working at cross-purposes. As Jacobson has noted, "the problems to be solved in the pursuit of the group objective seemed overwhelmed by the problems of working together" (Jacobson 1974, p. 753).

More questions about the purpose and nature of the study were raised by the committee members. They were probably reacting to the researcher's apparent ignorance or denial of their concerns. The decision to participate in developing a questionnaire was deferred while the nurses conducted a reconnaissance to other nursing services in their area and initiated contacts with various administrative departments within their own CMHC.

Finally, after several meetings, a consensus was reached by the researcher and the NSC that a questionnaire would be prepared by the nurses to be given to nurses. A meeting was held to generate ideas for the specific questions to be included, but only four committee members attended this special meeting, indicating that substantial resistance and mistrust had been building up during this phase. However, the researcher was confident that she could construct a questionnaire that would reflect the needs and thinking of the NSC. She planned to synthesize the suggestions of those at the meeting, other members' ideas and reactions as noted in the process recordings of prior meetings, and what she had learned from individual interviews. The researcher also investigated the nursing and community mental health literature to review the concepts and perceptions of the role of the psychiatric nurse as a guide in formulating the questions.

From these sources the researcher made a preliminary draft of a questionnaire to submit for the NSC's comments, revisions, and approval. She hoped that this tentative questionnaire would help to stimulate more discussion among the members and arouse enthusiasm for the project. The response she received from the committee was even more than she had bargained for.

The sixty-four questions devised by the researcher included a potpourri of items; some of them were of only peripheral interest to the nurses, but she had considered them potentially useful or interesting. However, once again the nurses perceived the researcher as pursuing her own interests and not theirs; she had used outside references for the questions, and had gone "beyond the clients." The questionnaire became a focal point for discharging negative feelings, questioning the researcher's motives, and revealing deep-seated resentment and suspicion of misguided intentions. The nurses were correct in criticizing the questionnaire for being too complicated and with too few items that pertained to their main concern about the nurse's role and other related matters of the NSC. It was also possible that the very wording and format of the questions might be construed as threatening to a group that had just started to make its presence known in a complex bureaucratic system. Yet the researcher's intentions were not opposed to those of the nurses, or so she thought. In an effort to give more than had been asked, the researcher antagonized the nurses by appearing to ask questions that came from other sources and that they had never mentioned. The tenuous relationship between the researcher and the client came dangerously close to terminating with bad feelings on both sides.

In retrospect, the researcher discovered that she had made several mistakes that Wilson states are among the most common in action research. The first is the researcher's failure to recognize not only the anxiety aroused in the client by the need to seek help but the inevitable apprehension about an intrusive researcher, no matter how benevolent. This researcher also failed to take sufficient account of her own anxiety about the new venture of doing action research. The second mistake is the researcher's tendency to take over the decision-making process, thereby negating the collaborative aspect of the relationship. A third mistake is that the researcher entered the system at the wrong point. Unwittingly, she appeared to be a representative of the Graduate School of Nursing with which the NSC was at odds on certain issues of overlapping interests and authority. This problem emerged during the conflict over the questionnaire when the nurses voiced approval of the researcher as a person, but disapproval of the system with which she was associated. The fourth difficulty pertains to the researcher's unconscious motivations and interests. As Wilson warns, "the temptation to take omnipotent executive action with one's first 'group-patients' needs considerable effort of resistance" (1947, pp. 26–28).

The conflict engendered by the questionnaire produced a new feeling of cohesion among the committee members themselves. They were spurred on to new levels of initiative and productivity. There were more regular meetings, a higher attendance at meetings, and more outside meetings among members.

The NSC began to revise the questionnaire expressly without the researcher's presence or participation. When the committee had finished, they met with the researcher to negotiate a formal contract for further participation in the study. The researcher agreed to draw up a new questionnaire based on the committee's suggested revisions. By this time, the researcher had a clearer idea of the client's needs and how to help meet them, and the client felt assured that the researcher would contribute what was necessary and appropriate toward solving their problem. The collaborative relationship had an emotional distance, but the relationship was less ambiguous than before the conflict. The researcher had to cope with her feelings of isolation, but recognized the group's need for independence and autonomy.

After the researcher redesigned the questionnaire, the committee approved it. The members seemed favorably impressed and pleased with the results of their collaboration on this new questionnaire. The chairpersons wrote a cover letter. The nurses assumed responsibility for distributing and collecting the questionnaire to and from all nurses employed in the CMHC. Later, the committee members took an active part in some aspects of analyzing the data.

Phases IV and V: Utilization and Evaluation   According to Lazarsfeld, "trust will not make the client free if he does not know what to do with it" (1975, p. 42); hence, there is a gap between knowledge and recommendations. The phase of utilization tries to narrow that gap by having the researcher and the client make creative use of the action research findings. Research has shown that utilization is increased if clients participate actively in the development of the project, if they have good rapport with the researchers, if their responses to the developing findings are sought and heeded, and if particular components or aspects of the findings could be used according to agencies' needs, rather than having to accept or adopt a total package (Glaser and Taylor 1973, pp. 144–145).

Evaluation is the follow-up to all that has gone before. It could include the writing and publishing of the research process and findings. It should include additional dissemination of the research findings in the form of workshops, seminars, and special institutes that would permit greater utilization as well as clarification and reformulation of the findings. An evaluation should provide a detailed assessment of the reasons for success as well as failure of a project.

In this study, the researcher could not continue with the client during the utilization and evaluation phases. As anticipated, the NSC called a general staff meeting of all nurses to present the findings of their survey. The research findings were utilized to provide the basis for developing new procedures to increase safety on the hospital units, for starting continuing education programs for the nurses, and for further clarifying the nurse's role through written job descriptions. This meeting was the beginning of a new mandate for the NSC based on centerwide support of nurses seeking new directions in their roles as psychiatric nurses in the CMHC.

SUMMARY

Action research is a collaborative process for achieving social change in the organizations of a complex society. Those engaged in action research encounter all the familiar complications and obstacles of the more traditional types of research. In addition, certain difficulties arise from the very nature of the research and from the interaction and relationship of the researcher and the client system working together in the midst of a complex organizational setting. There is a criticism and resistance from other researchers and professionals who are anxious to maintain and protect the "pure" scientific method. There is also resistance from the clients themselves who both want a change and fear the ensuing process and consequences of change. Their opposition can be minimized through skillful interpersonal relations, their participation in the decision-making process, and a realistic hope for an expeditious resolution to their problem.

In choosing to do action research, the nurse-researcher opts for the chance to make a real impact by virtue of a deeper commitment to clients who will ultimately share the benefits of the planned change that was geared to their own problem.

REFERENCES

Andreoli, Kathleen G.; and Thompson, Carole E. 1977. The nature of science in nursing. *Image* 9,2:32–37.

Argyris, Chris. 1970. *Intervention theory and method: a behavioral science view.* Reading, Mass.: Addison-Wesley.

Breu, Christine; and Dracup, Kathleen. 1976. Implementing nursing research in a critical care setting. *Journal of Nursing Administration* 6:14–17.

Cunningham, Bart. 1976. Action research: toward a procedural model. *Human Relations* 29,3:215–238.

Foster, Michael. 1972. An introduction to the theory and practice of action research in work organizations. *Human Relations* 25,6:529–556.

Glaser, Edward M.; and Taylor, Samuel H. 1973. Factors influencing the success of applied research. *American Psychologist* 28,2:140–146.

Gortner, Susan R.; Bloch, Doris; and Phillips, Thomas P. 1976. Contributions of nursing research to patient care. *Journal of Nursing Administration* 6,2:22–27.

Hirschowitz, Ralph G. 1974. Small group methods in the promotion of change within interagency networks: leadership models. In *The group as agent of change,* ed. Alfred Jacobs and Wilford W. Spradlin. New York: Behavioral Publications, pp. 228–251.

Jacobson, Sylvia. 1974. A study of interprofessional collaboration. *Nursing Outlook* 22,12:751–755.

King, Imogene M. 1976. The health care system: nursing intervention subsystem. In *Health research: the systems approach,* ed. Harriet H. Werley, Ann Zuzich, Myron Zajkowski, and A. Dawn Zagornik. New York: Springer, pp. 51–60.

Lazarsfeld, Paul F.; and Reitz, Jeffrey G. 1975. *An introduction to applied sociology.* New York: Elsevier.

Rapoport, Robert N. 1970. Three dilemmas in action research. *Human Relations* 23,6:499–513.

Rogers, Martha E. 1970. *An introduction to the theoretical basis of nursing.* Philadelphia: Davis.

Shea, Carole A. 1976. Action research with nurses in a community mental health center: a descriptive study. Master's thesis, Rutgers University.

Treece, Eleanor Walters; and Treece, James William, Jr. 1973. *Elements of research in nursing.* St. Louis: Mosby.

Wilson, A. L. M. 1947. Some implications of medical practice and social casework for action research. *Journal of Social Issues* 3:11–28.

Chapter 17

Working Committees

Kathy Hartnett

OBJECTIVES

After studying this chapter, the learner will:

- Define a working committee
- Define participative management
- Tell how a working committee should function
- Tell how a committee chairperson should function

INTRODUCTION

Since the 1950s there have been many changes in the way nursing services are organized. Since nursing services have become too complex for one person to direct, committees have been formed to accomplish the various tasks of the nursing organization. A committee is defined as a relatively stable group that meets periodically for a specific purpose and has some mechanism for recommending or implementing its decisions (Stevens

1975, p. 14). Committees are an organization's way to create and promote changes. In this chapter, the nature and complexities of the working committee will be fully outlined, and it is hoped that nurses will serve in a more informed and effective capacity on committees from here on.

A working committee is made up of nursing service members who help to accomplish the necessary work more effectively (Ganong 1972, p. 53). Committee members are staff nurses, nurse-managers, and nurse clinicians who have been chosen to sit on a committee because of their interest in improving the quality of nursing care and because of their ability to listen and solve problems. Examples of working committees include coordinating, nursing care, and staff development committees. For each committee the nature, authority, and membership should be clearly defined. Each committee may have an overlapping area of responsibility, but each contributes to the goals of the nursing services. The objectives of the nursing services must also contribute to the overall goals of the health care organization.

With working committees, the nursing-management process becomes more humanistically oriented, recognizing the dignity and potentialities of all individuals (Ganong 1972, p. 57). Certain tasks are delegated to the committee members, and they are encouraged to develop their leadership skills. Nurses need to get used to the idea that their input is desired and that the chairperson of the committee really wants their contribution to help achieve better nursing care (Ganong 1972, p. 57).

In some nursing organizations, committee membership is an expected part of every nurse's job; in others, membership is voluntary. Nurses may participate on committees to improve the nursing care on their respective units, or they may become members of more generalized working committees such as the coordinating or nursing care committees. The average size of a working committee is around ten members and they meet as often as needed to accomplish their purposes.

The concept of the working committee developed from the principles of participative management as described by McGregor (1970). He studied organizations and found that there were two prevailing views on employees. Theory Y holds that the average worker is someone who has the potential for more responsibility and leadership. This viewpoint corresponds with participative management and systems theory. Theory X, on the other hand, claims that the average worker has to be coerced in order for him to cooperate with the organizational objectives. This viewpoint often prevailed in factories and hospitals of the past.

Participative management is based on democratic principles that call for the superior and the subordinate to share in the goal-setting and decision-making processes (DiVicenti 1972, p. 73). Although decisions are ultimately made by the superior, subordinates participate in the analysis of the problem and propose a solution for its resolution. This method of management requires a sense of mutual trust and cooperation between the two groups. The organizational climate must not be threatened by participative methods and must be receptive to the group's attempt to create a positive change in the system. For this type of management to work, all participants need to learn about management and participative techniques. Inservice education programs on participative management can pave the way for the acceptance of this approach.

SYSTEMS THEORY AND THE COMMITTEE CONCEPT

Working committees need to utilize the open systems model in order to be most effective. Open systems move in the direction of differentiation and elaboration. The content and process of a committee should never be static but should be constantly developing. To maintain its openness, a committee needs to take in more energy from its environment than it expends. Channels must be open so that nonmembers of the committee can bring their concerns to the committee's attention. The committee should then analyze the members' problem and propose a solution to the problem. Feedback to the nonmembers of the committee must also be established either by a liaison from the committee or by calling a general staff meeting. The staff can then express their opinions on the committee's progress and present ideas for resolving or studying other problems.

The principle of equifinality holds that a system can reach the same final state from differing initial conditions and by a variety of paths (Katz 1966, p. 100). Committee members have different levels of expertise and experience, which increases the likelihood of more creative committee decisions. Individual differences among the committee members are seen as positive factors that contribute to the purpose of the committee, which is the pooling of knowledge and judgment.

Synergy is defined as the ability of organizational structures to destroy the polarity between selfishness and unselfishness on the part of the individuals who make up the organization (Jehring 1972, p. 38). Groups with high levels of synergy are more cohesive and able to share in the goal achievement. Synergy, however, cannot be reached quickly since people require time and opportunity to develop trust, communication, and commitment (DiVicenti 1972, p. 249).

Committees fail to be effective when they become a closed system. This happens when a committee focuses too intently on its internal organization and loses sight of its relationship to the total organizational environment. A state of entropy (being run down) occurs if the committee stops taking in information from the environment. The committee members could become distrustful of the administration and could actually work against the overall organizational goals. An environment that is characterized by distrust and anxiety will reduce the amount of information flow and cause people to block out, screen, or distort communication (Bailey 1975, p. 100).

FUNCTIONS OF WORKING COMMITTEES

The major function of any committee is coordination. Information is transmitted both upward to the top management and downward to the general staff. Minutes of each meeting are kept and members should receive copies of these minutes several days before the following committee meeting. An agenda should also be included so that members can prepare in advance for the discussions. Minutes should also be sent to the top management so that they can be informed of the committee's progress toward its goals.

Members of the committee may serve as liaison to other committees within the organization and to the staff on specific units. The liaison can provide information on the committee's objectives and bring suggestions back to the committee for consideration. A liaison may also be sent to the committee from the administration so that both sides can present their viewpoints on a problem.

Coordination among the working committees within the nursing services is critical to the effective operation of the nursing services. A linking pin system of committees works well so long as each committee does its work. If one committee is poorly organized, it may affect the functioning of another committee. Each committee could send a liaison to another nursing committee so that there would be an exchange of information between the two committees. This approach also keeps each committee on its toes.

Another function of committees is to advise. If a committee has a particular problem that it wishes to solve, the members may set out to collect data and analyze the findings. The findings are then formulated into specific goals and presented to the top management as recommendations. The top management then decides whether to implement the recommendations. It is important for the advisory committee to have the power to advise and to receive feedback from top management if its recommendations are turned down.

Some committees develop policies. Members of the organization work together to develop and revise policies for the organization. A bylaws committee is an example of a policy-making committee. Once the bylaws have been completed, the board of directors votes on them; if approved, the bylaws are then voted on by the staff. The bylaws then become the modus operandi of the organization since they contain the goals and functions of the various parts of the organization.

A committee may also provide a service. A nursing services committee, for example, could be organized to perform the functions of a director of nursing. Specific tasks and responsibilities would be delegated to the committee members so that the nursing services work could be done.

The functions of a committee will vary according to its goals. Organizations commonly utilize standing and task force committees to carry out certain essential functions. Standing committees are formally authorized and deal with policies, procedures, and research. Periodic status reports are sent to the administration to inform them of the committees' progress. Task force committees are designed to study a certain problem area. Each committee exists until its task is completed and then it is dissolved.

ADVANTAGES OF WORKING COMMITTEES

Longest claims that the biggest advantage of committees may be the increased motivation and commitment that come from participation (Longest 1976, p. 195). There is less resistance to change if nurses have participated in the planning and implementing of the change. There is a heightened sense of morale and the group's productivity gradually increases. Individuals evaluate themselves more highly because of their performance and there is greater job satisfaction because they are working together to improve nursing care.

Nurses develop more of a collegial relationship with one another, and they realize the importance of pooling their resources to enhance their problem-solving abilities. A committee allows a workload to be distributed so that committee members are responsible for certain tasks. Individuals feel a greater sense of autonomy and accountability in performing certain tasks for the committee. There are substantially fewer conflicts among committee members because they are able to communicate and clarify points of view. Lastly, with participation in nursing management, the turnover rate is lower and there is more harmony among nurses (Alexander 1972, p. 209).

DISADVANTAGES OF WORKING COMMITTEES

The most common criticisms of committees are that they are time consuming and expensive. Time is wasted if the committee's task is not clearly defined and if the members do not have enough knowledge and expertise to carry out their responsibilities on the committee. Committees are expensive if they are improperly run and if the members are primarily from the more highly paid levels of management. Members from the middle management and staff levels are less expensive to utilize, and they can often reach the same level of achievement as top management personnel. A divided level of responsibility may lead certain committee members to avoid getting down to work and to "pass the buck" if the committee is nonproductive.

A further disadvantage occurs when a committee becomes a power base for some of its members. One example is when sides are drawn on a crucial issue and the dominant side attempts to steamroller its point of view over the less powerful members. This is just the opposite of the advantage that can be achieved by integrated group judgment and the pooling of specialized knowledge (Longest 1976, p. 194).

Wright states that a committee is only as strong as the chairperson who is appointed (Wright 1972, p. 55). Some chairpersons may rely on the committee's decisions to avoid their own responsibility in taking decisive action. This situation could lead to prolonged discussions and watered-down decisions by the members.

SOURCES OF RESISTANCE AND HOW THEY CAN BE OVERCOME

Committee membership may be required in certain organizations, and nurses may react to this obligation by being passive-aggressive or passive-resistant. Indications of resistance include poor attendance, lack of enthusiasm for assigned tasks, lateness to meetings, fighting, and non-participation.

Three of the most common group problems that apply to committees as well are: conflict, apathy, and nonparticipation (Bradford 1976, p. 133). Conflicts may arise because members feel that the tasks they have been given are beyond their capacity or because members are loyal to outside groups that pose a conflicting interest. The group leader should encourage members to express their feelings toward the group task and point out what he or she thinks is happening among members to cause dissension. Group members should be reminded that the committee's objective is to engage all members in its work and to get a consensus of their judgments on the task at hand. Those who feel that they do not have the knowledge necessary for the committee's work can be encouraged to remain in the group, and a consultant can be brought in to help the group learn more about their area of focus.

Apathy occurs when the members do not think that the problem being worked on is important and when they would prefer to work on another problem. Sometimes members feel powerless to affect the final decision or feel that the decision will not produce the hoped-for change (Bradford 1976, p. 138). In some groups, prolonged fights have dominated the content of the meetings. The group leader should point out these obstacles and encourage members to listen to one another and be less partisan in their opinions. Group members should be reminded that diversity of opinions can lead to a more innovative decision. If members feel that the group decisions will have little effect on the administration, the group should examine its relationship with other groups that have power in the organization. The group may have to use confrontation and compromise tactics to help move into a position of strength.

Inadequate decision making occurs when a group has little cohesiveness and little confidence in its ability to make a decision. Any group needs time to develop a sense of trust and commitment to goals. There may be pressure upon the group to make a decision when not enough time has been allowed to work out a satisfactory solution. Pressure may be exerted because of administrative deadlines or because of peer pressure to side with a certain opinion-maker. The group leader should prevent rushed or slipshod decisions by postponing the vote and asking for more discussion on the issue. Randall suggests that proponents might speak on both sides of an issue and then members might place their opinions on record (Randall 1961, pp. 35–38). This method would encourage individual responses and responsibility in the deliberations. Sometimes a group cannot terminate its discussion on an issue. In this case, the group leader could pool the opinions of the group and then make a decision for the group.

Stevens claims that most resistance occurs because of misinformation and that opposition could be reduced simply by having an informational campaign in which a change and its implications for the personnel could be described briefly (Stevens 1977, p. 29). When dealing with resistance, it is important to be aware of the attitudes and behavior of the group members. The group leader should try to create a positive attitude toward the new idea so that the change will be more acceptable. If the resistance to change continues, the leader should introduce new information for the group's consideration. However, if this attempt fails, the leader must decide whether to shelve the change for a future time or force the change on the group and see what happens. It is not always possible for a change to be approved by group members before it is introduced, and the leader may have to insist on the change. In such a case, however, the change should be extremely important for fulfilling the organization's goals.

COMMITTEE LEADERSHIP AND DECISION MAKING

Stogdill defines a leader as one who acquires status through active participation in a group by demonstrating the capacity to carry cooperative tasks through to completion (Stogdill 1974, p. 65). The leader focuses heavily on team building and maintaining morale. There needs to be an element of mutual stimulation between the leader and the group if the group's goals are to be achieved (Yura 1976, p. 114). The leader attempts to influence the activities of the group toward establishing and achieving its goals. The leader's encouragement results in each member feeling that he or she is an essential part of the group effort (Yura 1976, p. 114).

Participative leadership calls for group participation in the problem-solving process, although the leader makes the decision. A leader needs to be able to take the initiative and assume responsibility; these qualities distinguish the leader from the other group members (Longest 1976, p. 196). The leader may delegate certain responsibilities to the committee such as setting short- and long-range goals, but the leader still needs to give his or her approval. Longest reports that in an analysis of eighteen studies on organizational change, it was found that successful changes used a shared approach, that is, superiors sought the participation of subordinates in the decision making. The leader, however, has the final voice in what decision is made.

Decision making is one of the most complex activities of a committee; it consists of the following stages: (1) identifying the problem, (2) enumerating the alternative solutions, (3) evaluating the alternatives, (4) selecting the best alternative, (5) implementing this solution, and (6) evaluating the outcome (Plachy 1976, p. 62). This process takes considerable time, and the leader needs to direct the committee members through the various stages. One technique for facilitating problem-solving is brainstorming. Judgment is suspended while the group members express their thoughts on a particular problem and offer tentative solutions. The leader can then summarize the group's thoughts. Taylor found that when groups used brainstorming, they came up with more ideas of better quality than would normally be the case with individuals (Taylor 1958).

The committee's decisions and achievements should be evaluated on a regular basis. These activities are often incorporated in an annual report, and this is one way for top management to review whether a committee should continue to exist.

CLINICAL EXAMPLE

A nursing services committee within a community mental health center coordinated the nursing services provided through the operating units of the center. It was responsible for establishing standards for high quality nursing care, developing policies and procedures, reviewing the training needs of the staff nurses, and developing the training programs. The committee was designed as an advisory committee and was to report its progress and recommendations to the director of the center.

In this community mental health center, there were no directors of the professional groups. Each discipline—psychology, social work, medicine, and nursing—had its own service committee, and each committee elected a chairperson for a one-year term. The nursing services committee was composed of eleven members who were appointed by the director for one year. Meetings were to be held at least once a month, and the minutes were to be sent to the director.

During the nursing services committee's second year, it focused on goals. Two short-term goals were established without much disagreement: development of job descriptions for all the nurses and an orientation manual for new nurses. Individual members of the committee took responsibility for coordinating these tasks. The larger and more difficult matter of setting long-term goals was complicated by differences of opinion on the nursing leadership. Some committee members felt that there should be a director of nurses who would take full responsibility for organizing the nursing services, and others felt that the nursing services committee should continue its coordinating role as originally planned. Since the committee could not resolve this difference, it continued with its short-range goals and focused on problems.

The leadership of the committee changed during the second year. Two members of the committee were elected to share the leadership role. One chairperson was to coordinate the inhouse nursing organization, and the other was to coordinate the nursing organization on community teams. Their first project was to hold a general meeting of staff nurses to learn what their concerns were. They found that the nurses were troubled about the oncall system, safety factors on the nursing units, inservice education, salary, and tuition reimbursement.

The nursing services committee undertook an analysis of the existing situations and then proposed solutions to these problems. The committee found that the administration and personnel departments were responsive to about half of their requests. The administration sent a liaison person to the committee, which helped to open up communication between the two groups. The head of the personnel department was willing to discuss salary negotiations and tuition reimbursements with the committee but wanted to keep the information as secret as possible. Salary increments finally did go through, but tuition reimbursements were not feasible at that time.

During that period, a graduate student in a university-affiliated

psychiatric nursing program asked to attend a meeting of the nursing services committee with the idea of possibly planning a research project with
the committee. She wanted to do an action-research project and offered to
help the committee study one of its areas of interest. The committee decided to develop a questionnaire to elicit the opinions of nurses within the
community mental health center on morale, role models, and whether the
current committee leadership was preferable to having a director of
nurses. The questionnaire was drafted by the committee and the researcher and then distributed to all of the nurses within the nursing services; 78 percent of them answered the questionnaire. The results showed
that 67 percent wanted a director of nurses to take responsibility for the
nursing leadership; about half the nurses had high morale and half had low
morale; and the majority of nurses had no role models (Shea 1976, pp.
95–98). It appeared that the nursing services committee had very little
influence within the community mental health center, and the majority of
nurses felt that the committee needed more power; they also suggested
having more regular nursing staff meetings.

The committee then presented these questionnaire results to the administration. It was not possible to hire a director of nursing because of
budgetary restrictions. The committee decided to have one chairperson
and to expand the role for the forthcoming year. The chairperson would
sit on the important organizational committees as nursing's representative, and she would have free time during the work week to devote to the
task of nursing organization. This idea was presented at a general meeting
of staff nurses and was approved.

By the end of the second year, the nursing services committee had a
clearer idea of its direction. The committee members felt a sense of accomplishment in that they had resolved certain bothersome questions.
There was a higher level of cohesion and more members shared in the
committee's communications. The members felt more confident about
continuing to work with the committee, and they were more knowledgeable about how to make the committee responsive to the work environment. The members realized that they needed to have more contacts
within the administration in order to build up their power in the organization.

In retrospect, the nursing services committee utilized the
participative-management approach but without having a strong
decision maker. The committee learned to manage by doing it. Inservice
education programs on participative management would have been helpful to improve the members' competence. However, the committee members worked collaboratively to improve the nursing services and they
learned how a committee has to relate to the entire system in order to
function effectively. As a result, the morale of the committee members

increased greatly, and they became interested in developing their leadership skills. The committee members had matured through their experience on the committee, and they were looking forward to the future development of the nursing services committee.

SUMMARY

A working committee is composed of nursing service members who work together to accomplish the necessary work more effectively. The functions of working committees are to coordinate, advise, develop policies, and provide services. Common group problems that impede the work of committees are conflict, apathy, and nonparticipation. Participative leadership calls for group participation in the problem-solving process. One example of a working committee was described—a nursing services committee within a community mental health center.

REFERENCES

Alexander, Edythe. 1972. *Nursing administration in the hospital care system.* St. Louis: Mosby.

Bailey, June; and Claus, Karen. 1975. *Decision making in nursing—tools for change.* St. Louis: Mosby.

Bradford, Leland; Stock, Dorothy; and Horwitz, Murray. 1976. How to diagnose group problems. In *Management for nurses: a multidisciplinary approach,* ed. Sandra Stone et al. St. Louis: Mosby.

Cooper, Signe. 1973. Committees that work. *Journal of Nursing Administration* 3,1:30–35.

DiVicenti, Marci. 1972. *Administering nursing service.* Boston: Little, Brown.

Ganong, Warren; and Ganong, Joan Mary. 1972. Reducing organizational conflict through working committees. *Journal of Nursing Administration* 2,1:12–19.

Hill, Barbara Snyder. 1976. Participative management: a valid alternative to traditional organizational behavior. *Supervisor Nurse* 7,3:19–21.

Jehring, J. J. 1972. Motivational problems in the modern hospital. *Journal of Nursing Administration* 2,6:35–41.

Katz, D.; and Kahn, R. L. 1969. Common characteristics of open systems. In *Systems thinking,* ed. F. E. Emery. Baltimore: Penguin, pp. 86–104.

Likert, R. 1967. *The human organization, its management and values.* New York: McGraw-Hill.

Longest, Beaufort. 1976. *Management practices for the health professional.* Reston, Va.: Reston Publishing.

McGregor, D. 1970. *The human side of enterprise.* New York: McGraw-Hill.

Plachy, Roger. 1976. Delegation and decision making. In *Management for nurses: a multidisciplinary approach,* ed. Sandra Stone et al. St. Louis: Mosby, pp. 58–65.

Randall, C. 1961. *The folklore of management.* Boston: Little, Brown.

Shea, Carole A. 1976. Action research with nurses in a community mental health center: a descriptive study. Master's thesis, Rutgers University.

Stevens, Barbara. 1975. *The nurse as executive.* Wakefield, Mass.: Contemporary.

———. 1977. Management of continuity and change in nursing. *Journal of Nursing Administration* 7,4:26–31.

Stogdill, R. 1974. *Handbook of leadership.* New York: Free Press.

Taylor, D.; Berry, P. C.; and Block, C. H. 1958. Does group participation when using brainstorming facilitate or inhibit creative thinking? *Administrative Science Quarterly* 3:23–47.

Wright, Nadian E. 1972. How central service supervisor can contribute to work of key hospital committees. *Hospital Topics* 50,6:55–57.

Yura, Helen; Ozmiak, Dorothy; and Walsh, Mary. 1976. *Nursing leadership theory and process.* New York: Appleton-Century-Crofts.

Chapter 18

Self-Management and Nursing

Ruth R. Greenberg Edelstein

OBJECTIVES

After studying this chapter, the learner will:

- Define self-management
- Give the rationale for self-management
- Explain how self-management fits into systems theory
- Describe the origins of the self-management movement
- Give examples of self-management in practice
- Enumerate ways in which self-management may be applied in health care services
- Point out pseudo forms of participation
- Explain how nurses may be viewed as members of the new working class and how this relates to self-management
- Discuss the role of unions in self-management
- List certain problems in instituting self-management
- Discuss the possibilities of instituting self-management in nursing practice

WHAT IS SELF-MANAGEMENT?

Self-management is the control of working time by those who do the work. It is the participation of all of those who work in an enterprise in the basic decisions of its operation. Self-management relates to nurses because they are deeply concerned about how they spend their time at work and how the health care system operates. They are also concerned about working conditions as one of the major environmental factors influencing their clients. Like their clients, nurses often spend an inordinate amount of time in meaningless and dehumanizing activities. Many find themselves in work situations where they have little or no control over what happens.

Most Europeans have their own terms for workplace democracy such as "workers' control," "industrial democracy," "Mitbestimmung," "autogestion," and "self-management." Except for "autogestion" and "self-management," the other expressions usually refer to participatory schemes that fall far short of self-management. In the United States the terms "self-management" and "workers' control" are relatively unknown. "Although the reforms being promoted vary from country to country, they have one point in common: the transfer of real decision-making power to employees" (Jenkins 1974, p. 15).

WHY SELF-MANAGEMENT?

Self-management in health care organizations means that the health workers determine the goals of the organization and how they shall be achieved, and they implement the plans they have made. "Self-management . . . does away with that division of labor which is essentially identical to the division of society into two basic classes, i.e., the minority of leaders and the majority of those who execute orders" (Goricar 1972, p. 18). "Its essential characteristic . . . is the exclusive control and management of productive organizations by [their] *full* active membership on a basis of equality of vote" (Vanek 1975, p. 14). Self-management is based on a libertarian model of social organization that emphasizes participatory democracy but goes beyond it.

Self-management principles assume that (1) all people seek and need responsibility; (2) imagination, ingenuity, and creativity are widely distributed among the population; (3) modern working conditions generally impair the realization of the individual's potentialities; (4) democracy pertains not only to a government but to a social system; and (5) the perception of self-worth should be distributed evenly throughout the population (Supek 1972, p. 173; Garson 1972, pp. 89, 108).

SYSTEMS CONTEXT OF SELF-MANAGEMENT

Self-management is active participation in the development of a self-organizing system (McEwan 1971, p. 179). Self-management pertains to the democratic nature of systems; an opposite characteristic of systems —symbolic pseudo participation—keeps an existing system at the same level with very little development.

Self-management encourages self-organizing systems since it deemphasizes role assignments and stereotyped procedures. A system that is not self-managing does not work well. The reason committees sometimes have difficulty making good decisions is not the group process per se but the role assignments and stereotyped procedures that restrict its development. Outside higher committees, which establish rules and procedures in a particular work situation, are necessarily occupied with standard procedures and rigid structures. The information available at the top echelon is inherently inadequate. Those in charge have to make innumerable rules, but the more the rules take account of every possible event that might occur, the more stymied are those who are trying to get a job done. If these people actually followed all of the rules, they would be paralyzed (this happens when "working to rule" is invoked as a weapon in a labor dispute) (McEwan 1971, p. 187).

In a model of pyramidal hierarchy, there is fixed delineation of responsibility, procedures are narrowly outlined, and a change can be made only by those at the highest level of the hierarchy where the "brain" of the system is alleged to sit. An alternate model of management is "characterized by a changing structure that modifies itself under continual feedback from the environment, exhibits redundancy of potential command, and involves complex interlocking control structures. The 'brain' is distributed throughout the system" (McEwan 1971, p. 188). Harmony is sought in an "ever changing and fugitive equilibrium of varied forces and influences of every kind, following their own course" (McEwan 1971, p. 189).

ORIGINS OF THE MOVEMENT

The self-management movement had its origins in England and France. The idea originated early in the nineteenth century with Buchez (Phillippe-Joseph-Baptiste Buchez), a French medical doctor as well as a philosopher, historian, and journalist who wanted to put "Christianity into practice." For him this meant putting democracy into people's everyday work as well as the government. Toward this goal, he advocated a "workingman's association" that "would be based on the accumulation of a stock of 'social, inalienable capital' contributed by the members [that would become] the permanent property of the association and a guarantee of its perpetuity'' (Vanek 1975, p. 17).

The Robert Owen-inspired Pioneers of Rochdale in England, set up in 1844, is the forerunner of some of the earlier and current efforts at self-management through the formation of cooperatives. An entire city was organized around the concept of autonomous, decentralized units and workers' self-management (the Paris Commune, which lasted from March to May 1871, "when it was brutally crushed") (Vanek 1975, p. 19). "Works councils," which were organized from above in Germany in the 1890s, "gave workers some small measure of codetermination along with management and entrepreneurs" (Vanek 1975, p. 20).

Various types of communes organized around the idea of equality at the place of work were tried abortively in the United States in the last century. In 1840, George Ripley, together with a group of twenty persons (including Nathaniel Hawthorne) set up the Brook Farm Institute for Agriculture and Education at West Roxbury, near Boston. They wanted to substitute "a system of brotherly (sisterly) cooperation for one of selfish competition . . . to institute an attractive, efficient, and productive system of industry . . . to guarantee . . . physical support and spiritual progress, and thus to impart a greater freedom, simplicity, truthfulness, refinement, and moral dignity to . . . life" (Hillquit 1903, p. 96). This experiment, which followed the ideas of the French utopian socialist Charles Fourier, prospered for a number of years.

SELF-MANAGEMENT IN CURRENT PRACTICE

A wide range of structural arrangements aimed at some form of workplace democracy are proving functional in Europe, Israel, and the United States. Democratization of the workplace has become a key issue for European unions. It has been supported by the European Economic Community (Employee Participation and Company Structure in the European Community 1975, p. 10). In several countries national legislation has assured the enactment of some form of workers' participation in all enterprises of any size (West Germany, Scandinavia, the Netherlands, Yugoslavia). A wide range of findings from efforts at self-management have implications for self-management in the health care industry, as well as for the quality of life and the status of health.

The kibbutzim in Israel are almost totally self-managed; 230 kibbutzim (groups) are owned and operated by 90,000 members. These are both residential communities and places of work. They differ from other self-management enterprises in that the members have close ties in all aspects of their life together (Jenkins 1974, pp. 73–75).

No one living in a kibbutz has to worry about the cost of food, rent, or health care. Health care, whether given at the kibbutz or in a hospital, is paid for by the kibbutz. If necessary, the kibbutz arranges for special care. There is no unemployment. The old, the sick, and the disabled are completely provided for (Spiro 1970, pp. 86–87).

In the work situation, all those who hold managerial positions are elected. Policy decisions are made by the workers, and most jobs are rotated (Spiro 1970, p. 82). The welfare of the group depends upon the industriousness of the individual members. Everyone is aware that the living standards of each person depend upon the united efforts of all. The kibbutzim demonstrate the viability and endurability of a democratic system of self-management that unites work and life (Jenkins 1974, pp. 83–84, 90–91).

Yugoslavia has a system of self-management that applies to every enterprise in the country. All workers are either members of a workers' council, or they elect representatives to such a council in enterprises that employ more than thirty persons. In turn, the council selects members of the managing board and appoints management personnel. Managerial decisions must be approved by the council. The council is also responsible for salary scales, hiring and firing, investment programs, and long-term planning. "Salaries are based on a base pay plus an additional amount determined by the company's 'profits'" (Jenkins 1974, pp. 96, 101). In most cases the workers in Yugoslavia receive much more information about the financial and operational data of their firm than do workers in Britain and the United States (Kolaja 1965, p. 60).

No other West European country has gone as far as West Germany in formalizing employee participation in management. In 1951 the Codetermination Act was passed for the coal and steel industries, requiring worker representatives to constitute half of the board of directors. In 1952 the Works Constitution Act established works councils in all enterprises where there are more than five workers and required one-third representation of labor on all boards of directors except in the coal and steel industries (Bye 1973, p. 5).

The unions generally believe that these advances are too limited, and they are disappointed that the parity achieved in the coal and steel industries has not been obtained elsewhere (Elvin 1976). In 1976 West Germany passed legislation giving employees 50 percent representation on the board of directors, but this parity was spoiled by the stipulation that one of the employees must be from top management (Elvin 1976). American-based multinationals situated in West Germany feel threatened by these industrial arrangements (*when workers help call the time in management* 1976, p. 83). The unions are anxious to keep the gains they have made, and they hope to establish more parity in various enterprises in the future.

In the United States and England attempts to establish self-managed enterprises have been made primarily in private cooperatives. The highly successful worker-owned plywood mills in the western United States consist of twenty manufacturing cooperatives. Their principles of organization are as follows: "Each owner has only one vote regardless of the number of shares he holds; income or surplus is returned to the owners as workers and as dividends on capital; available work is distributed among all owners who wish to work; all worker-owners receive the same hourly wage rate; final authority resides in a general meeting of the membership" (Bellas 1974, pp. 205–206).

SELF-MANAGEMENT AND HEALTH CARE

Self-management has been tried in mental hospitals These attempts were planned as treatment methods appropriate to the needs of the clients. Some of their major limitations related to the emphasis on treatment; little or no consideration was given to industrial democracy for the workers at the institution. An early advocate of self-management in health care was Maxwell Jones of the Henderson Hospital in England. He engaged the clients in decision-making processes during their hospital stay and minimized the role distinctions within the hospital (Jones 1953). To accomplish this, common goals had to be established, power decentralized, avenues of communication opened, and responsibility given to clients. Therefore, the traditional relationship between treater and treated was changed considerably (Abrahamsson 1973, p. 178).

Ward attendants were the most resistant to the normative standards of the therapeutic communities in psychiatric hospitals in Britain and France. This resistance tended to be viewed as personal or due to recalcitrance or a lack of ability. A British solution was to replace the attendants with low-paid university graduates (Jones 1973, pp. 167–168).

One obvious point was that the therapeutic community was initiated at the top of the hierarchy, usually with psychiatrists. Little consideration was given to the fact that attendants were evaluated and promoted by chief attendants who placed great value on orderliness and "proper control" of the clients, criteria that were given low priority in the therapeutic community. When the client role was redefined, giving the patient the right to refuse to work, an additional work burden fell on the attendants. "It would appear that the attendants were expected to participate in decisions on matters previously thought to be beyond them, and their control over the patients, seen as critical in relation to the evaluation of attendants' performances, was weakened" (Jones 1953, p. 186).

In a Finnish hospital Kock found that such features as cooperation, job involvement, openness to change, and flexibility of the ward staff were related to a less formal communication, less social distance, and greater group orientation on the part of the head nurse. It would appear that, even within a hierarchical setting, certain individuals can foster more democratic participation within their isolated units (Kock 1973).

Zahourek, Leone, and Lang set up a group nursing practice in Denver that had some of the earmarks of a self-management enterprise. "A core group of about ten people consistently attended meetings" before the group became incorporated (Zahourek et al. 1976, p. 26). At the beginning sixteen stockholders contributed $300 each, but only eight had plans to practice (Zahourek et al. 1976, p. 29). In December 1973 they established the Creative Health Services, a name selected by the group. The corporation stock that could be held by any one person was limited to 45 percent. A maximum of $50,000 worth of no par common stock was issued. The stockholders elected five directors on an annual basis, and the directors elected the officers (Zahourek et al. 1976, pp. 32–33).

The nurse "practitioners were paid on the basis of income generated and collected" (Zahourek et al. 1976, p. 35). Clerical work was budgeted for, and so the secretary did not fall into the stockholder-practitioner category but received a regular salary. However, the practitioners shared responsibility for covering the routine clerical and reception work when the secretary was not there. A "formation team" of practitioners and hired experts (an attorney and an accountant) were responsible for structuring the group practice in compliance with required regulations (Zahourek et al. 1976, 39).

The group was handicapped in trying to realize a more democratic structure because the practitioners all held other jobs as well, were not fully committed, and carried unequal burdens of the workload. The practitioners, as well as the stockholders, met very infrequently. "Each clinical specialty group met separately so that an exchange of ideas and stimulation between the groups occurred only sporadically" (Zahourek et al. 1976, p. 97).

The primary nursing care of the nurses at the Loeb Center for Nursing and Rehabilitation at Montefiore Hospital, Bronx, New York, has aspects of self-management built into it. The nurses have the freedom to practice their profession without interference from rigid hierarchical work structures. When the self-management movement takes root in health care institutions, it will probably start at centers such as this one.

A bill to establish a national community health service was introduced into Congress by Ronald Dellums of California in 1976. It emphasizes self-management by providing "health workers with opportunities for full and equal participation in the governance of health facilities; for advancement without regard to race, sex, age, national origin, religion, or political belief; and for fair and reasonable compensation and security" (Community Health Alternatives Project 1976, p. v). The bill provides for:

> . . . area health facilities to be managed by the workers on a democratic basis. Toward this end, each area health board shall develop and implement a plan for democratic decision making within each area health facility under its supervision, including mechanisms for full and equal participation of health workers at all skill levels (Community Health Alternatives Project, 1976).

Those who framed this proposal were so influenced by the professionals in the health care system that, despite their extreme commitment to participatory democracy, they specified that no health worker should be allowed to serve on the elected community health board. This is contrary to all attempts in industrial enterprises to give workers a place on governing boards.

RECOGNIZING PSEUDO PARTICIPATION TACTICS

While "the notion of participatory planning/decision making/governance is one that is widely accepted in this country . . . participatory planning as practiced in most American endeavors is honored either through crudely superficial devices, such as advisory councils or public opinion polls, or entirely in the breach" (Kaplan 1975, p. 2). The fact is that, regardless of the prevailing political institutions of a country, democratic participation in the economic enterprises is a problem.

Traditional management represents the power base of most institutions. Top-, middle-, and lower-level management cooperate together to retain this power base. Those currently sitting in seats of power are not about to abdicate or share their power without a struggle. The managers in West Germany did not allow the codetermination law to pass without a big fight.

Nurses, when they are managers, most often appear at the middle and lower levels of management (head nurses, supervisors, coordinators, and so forth) and are frequently responsible to a nonnurse who is the top manager. This makes nursing managers more sympathetic to the lower echelon, although their desire to maintain their administrative posts militates against acting on these sympathies. Management jobs have almost always entailed higher pay, supposedly greater responsibility, and greater allegiance to top management. Sometimes nurses in lower management have found themselves in a dilemma, torn between loyalty to the top management which can fire them and to the workers below with whom they sometimes feel aligned against top management. This dilemma is often brought about by what seem to be arbitrary or exploitative directives from above.

The centralization of decision making is fairly well recognized as inefficient in most institutions. Knowing this, administrators often make an effort to try to appear to be sharing the decision making. Such efforts are usually for show or done in the hope that they will relieve the tensions and malfunctions that result from autocratic rule.

Why does the development of participatory democracy come so hard? One reason is that organizations have usually operated by "setting a stage for the exercise of power" (Zaleznik 1976, p. 13). "The development of careers, particularly at high managerial and professional levels, depends on accumulation of power as the vehicle for transforming individual interests into activities which influence other people" (Zaleznik 1976, p. 14). However, a system built on centralized power leads to defective functioning very quickly. Traditional management views the resulting behaviors as evidence of personality conflicts, paranoid thinking, and the inability to be creative (Zaleznik 1976, p. 33). In accordance with the symptoms noted, management invents participatory games to cure people and to get them to fit the institutional mold better. "Social psychotherapy" sometimes is used for temporary relief of authoritariansim.

Zaleznik scoffs at some of the ritualistic uses of small groups that are often made by management to placate subordinates and to evade issues that challenge their authority. The participatory game has very little to do with libertarianism and democracy. Often groups meet away from work because someone thinks that tensions produced by competitive and inegalitarian work climates can be dissolved in this way. Such efforts usually result in temporary peace and feelings of well-being that are brought about by overindulgence in food and drink. Human relations programs and sensitivity training, like the feasts, attempt to convert the worker ideologically to management's schemes rather than to promote democracy at the workplace (Zaleznik 1976, p. 31).

Job redesign and profit sharing are palliative measures, and it depends how they are done whether they are pro-democratic or not. They do not add up to self-management. Full participation requires the institutionalization of self-management as an enterprisewide system of decision making.

THE NEW WORKING CLASS AND NURSES

To identify different classes within a society is to set up a framework for determining the nature of the relationships among the classes. Gorz, Mallet, Touraine, and others have recognized the existence of a new working class that includes white collar workers, various types of experts, teachers, research workers, professionals, and so forth (Gorz 1967; Mallet 1975; Touraine 1966). This class is characterized by: (1) higher education, (2) specialization, (3) job insecurity, (4) fear of competition, (5) dread of immobility, (6) identity uncertainty, and (7) dismay over the insignificance of one's life. Many members of the new working class lack class consciousness because they are so much a part of the prevailing system. Class consciousness is a prerequisite for mounting an active program to eliminate class differences and to establish self-management at the place of work.

Nurses educated at the associate, baccalaureate, master's, and doctoral degree levels tend to create their own pseudo class system. Ambivalent statuses and multiple allegiances characterize most workers who are not clearly members of the working class. Recognition of nursing's place in the new working class should help to clarify some of the confusion. The nurse's aides and attendants are his or her confederates in the "old" working class. The new working class "is the natural ally of the working class and the labor movement" (Denitch 1977, p. 70).

There is a social antimanual ethic that leads to rejection of collaboration with those who are members of the "old" working class. This comes from a more that mental work is more honorable and that those who have more leisure are of greater worth (Veblen 1953). Members of the new working class:

> . . . use many dodges to avoid identification with wage-workers and yet secure the benefits of unionism. They call their unions "guilds" or "associations"; they have a permanent no-strike policy, etc. In the end this is nonsense so far as the central economic purpose of unions is concerned; yet, although their sacrifice of prestige is the sacrifice of a fading value, this value is still real to white-collar employees, often more so than their low incomes (Mills 1953, pp. 312–313).

Nurses do not belong to the same class as physicians, who generally control their own work almost completely and earn at least six to seven times as much as nurses and often substantially more. Seldom are nurses able to carry out fully what they are capable of doing to improve the health care of clients. They have little control over the operation of the employing institution, even though formally they may have the opportunity to talk about it. The initial steps toward self-management must be the narrowing of differences between the classes that make up the health care system. For the new and the "old" working classes, this means increased participation in the major decisions that affect their working conditions.

The dependent status of the nurse of a century ago is incongruous today. Through restrictions on their freedom in a strictly hierarchical health care system, nurses cannot give the kind of comprehensive health care they are capable of giving. The gross discrepancy between status and capability are preconditions for revolt against the class system that keeps them in bondage.

WHAT IS THE ROLE OF UNIONS?

Unionism fits in with self-management, but self-management goes beyond unionism. The union contract protects the worker over a period of time, while self-management is a decision-making system at work. Through collective bargaining, nurses can establish contractual agreements that initiate self-management processes.

Some would have the unions continue their usual function of safeguarding the workers' rights and maintaining an independent role of outside watchdog even under self-management (Clegg 1960). However, others see unions as the major instrument for establishing and operating self-managed enterprises (Blumberg 1973, p. 83). For instance, in some countries (such as West Germany) the trade unions elect some of the workers' representatives to the boards of firms.

The American Nurses Association, a world pioneer in professional unionism, has successfully been able to reconcile professionalism with the use of collective bargaining. The professional component in unionism tends to place some emphasis on the "product," for example, stating that when nurses have poor working conditons, they give poor nursing care (Grand 1976, p. 261). But "productivity" is not the issue. Like all workers, nurses have the right to working conditions where they have control over real decision-making processes. Overemphasizing the quality of nursing care as a prime concern tends to cloud the issue of the rights of nurses as workers. Such emphasis leads some nurses to assume (erroneously) that it is "unprofessional" to be concerned about their own rights.

PROBLEMS IN SELF-MANAGEMENT

The greatest amount of empirical work on self-managed enterprises has been done by Yugoslavian sociologists. They have come up with evidence of a number of problems in establishing a self-management system. Some of the problems may be due to the fact that Yugoslavia has a one-party system of government and one might wonder how participatory democracy could function at work places in such a country. Nevertheless, the sociologists have been readily publishing their findings.

In reviewing the data, Warner found that some workers' councils initiate fewer decisions than top and middle management; that active participants in the self-management schemes sometimes felt more alienated than the nonparticipants; that top management, although it has less power than its counterparts in other countries, exerts a greater influence on the workers; that those with more education take a greater part in discussions; that specialists "contribute out of all proportion to their percentage of representation" (Warner 1974, pp. 4–6).

Under German codetermination, workers' participation is often illusory. Workers' representatives on the supervisory boards, even when they comprise half of the board membership, tend not to challenge management's power over technical matters. The workers' representatives leave investment policy and other issues to the experts and concentrate on questions of employment and conditions. They interfere "very little with the actual running of the place of work while giving the seal of respectability to management policies" (Bye 1973, p. 19)

In the plywood cooperatives in the United States, there is a tendency toward instability. One of the reasons for this is that there is an emphasis on maximization of current worker-owner income and a disregard for profits over a period of time. There is a conflict between maximum return for effort and the long-run survival of the firm. Without strategic reinvestments, firms cannot "achieve a stability or growth of income to the owners" (Bellas 1975, pp. 209–210).

The problem of status differentials is not easily resolved. There are experts, professionals, and those with greater knowledge and experience, and it is inevitable that these people are going to have more to say and a great deal more influence than workers with less education and training. Part of the answer may lie in the approach used by Fr. José Maria in Mondragon, Spain. In the 1950s, and despite the reign of the dictator Franco, he set up a number of cooperatives that are thriving today, employing about 10,000 people. Most significant, they have their own "hybrid educational institution that turns out both machine operatives and craftsmen, and engineers with degree qualifications" (Oakeshott 1975, pp. 290–291). Also, in Yugoslavia workers are given time out from work to go to school to learn management skills.

It is important that new, self-managed enterprises get competent assistance so that many problems can be avoided. Toward this end, the Federation for Economic Democracy was established with headquarters in Washington, D.C. It is geared to help self-managment enterprises get started and to provide education for work in self-managed organizations.

IS SELF-MANAGEMENT POSSIBLE IN NURSING PRACTICE?

Two factors that interfere significantly with the democratization of nursing practice are traditional professionalism and "scientific management."

Self-management needs a reformulation of the concept of professionalism. Traditional professionalism stands for: (1) specialization that leads to dominance in a division of labor, (2) management of clients from a particular frame of reference, (3) monopoly in a specific area of work, (4) monopoly in the evaluation of that work, and (5) claims that no others can perform certain complex skills (Friedson 1970, pp. xvii and 45).

If we redefine professionalism as "the ability to convey objectively components of a special body of knowledge and to demonstrate special skills," then it can fit into self-management. However, traditional professionalism—which aims at the monopoly of knowledge and the restriction of skilled operations to one group—is incompatible with self-management.

> The fundamental principle of "scientific management" is the concentration of decisions in the hands of a central authority. . . . [Nurses] no longer represent a highly skilled, diversely utilizable potentiality, but . . . [people] assigned to work posts. Task analysis does not concern itself with the individual potential of this or that worker, but with stages of the production process [patient-processing procedures] (Mallet 1975, p. 32).

Management has devised certain staffing methods that apply dehumanized industrial tactics to health care. These methods attempt to ascertain the smallest number nurses who can do the nursing care and the number of "nursing" tasks that can be done by unskilled workers. The staff nurse has very little, if any, voice in the decisions reached. The methods call for task and procedure analyses, classification of clients according to "needs," classification of "nursing" tasks according to time required, and the classification of these tasks according to cost (Aydelotte 1973, p. 46).

The mechanization of industrial workers is an unhealthy development for the workers, but the mechanization of a health care system adds insult to injury. However, it certainly is not an unexpected development in a society where the long-term trend is to simplify and deskill jobs to cut costs. "Translated into market terms, this means that the labor power capable of performing the process may be purchased more cheaply as dissociated elements than as a capacity integrated in a single worker" (Braverman 1974, p. 81).

Self-management in nursing is participation in the management of the health care enterprise by nurses. It refers to health care organizations in which those in managerial roles are no longer appointed but rather elected to terms of office. The elected managers carry out their work on the basis of policy decisions made by the nurses and others who work in the unit, department, hospital, and so forth. The development of goals and plans for evaluation of work are horizontal functions; there are no directives orginating from above and passed downward.

Although a full system of self-management in nursing would require democratization of the total health care system, there is evidence that self-management could be put into effect at local levels where there is enough enthusiasm, commitment, and dedication toward the establishment of an egalitarian system of health care. Health worker cooperatives and nursing centers are ideal settings for self-management ventures.

The place where self-management could probably best develop would be a libertarian health facility that emphasized a holistic health model with the view that: (1) individual illness is a reflection of social illness; (2) illness has multiple causes; (3) curative care is ultimately insufficient; (4) health care requires an active program of prevention; and (5) social restructuring is necessary to maintain acceptable levels of health (Hays-Bautista and Harveston 1977, pp. 8–9).

An intermediary step toward the democratization of the workplace that could be taken today at any health institution that has collective bargaining would be the negotiation of what the British call a "status quo agreement." This is an agreement between management and health workers that management will make no changes whatsoever that affect these workers without their prior agreement. It has been found that this agreement, contrary to what "status quo" implies, leads to greater flexibility in the organization and to mutually acceptable innovations. Workers tend to accept reasonable proposals when they have participated in the decision making (Whitty 1976).

THE CONSUMER AND NURSING SELF-MANAGEMENT

The essence of self-management is that the workers have the primary say in daily operations. However, service-oriented enterprises have different problems than industrial enterprises. Whereas in industry the product reaches a distant customer, in health services the "customer" is deeply involved in the work process itself. Therefore, community members and clients need to play some part in the management of nursing services.

Community spokespersons should be represented on all decision-making boards. Consumer participation on boards can easily be implemented; how they might participate in the daily operation of a nursing service is less clear and represents an area for creative, innovative ideas. One way in which consumers could participate directly in the daily operations of a health facility would be through part-time work assignments either as hospital clients or as community health aides.

SUMMARY

Self-management is the participation of all those who work in an enterprise in the basic decisions of its operation. It is based on a libertarian model of social organization that emphasizes participatory democracy but goes beyond it. It requires active participation in the development of an ongoing, self-organizing system.

The movement originated in France and England during the last century. A wide variety of structural arrangements aimed at some form of workplace democracy is being tried in Europe, Israel, and the United States. The best current examples of self-management are the kibbutzim in Israel.

In health care enterprises, the initial steps toward self-management would have to be the narrowing of differences among the classes that make up the health care system. Group nursing practices, health worker cooperatives, and nursing centers are ideal settings for self-management ventures. The place where it would be most likely to develop would be a libertarian health facility that emphasized a holistic health model. Through collective bargaining, nurses can establish contractual agreements that initiate self-management processes.

REFERENCES

Abrahamsson, B. 1972. Conditions for participation in treatment organizations. *First international sociological conference on participation and self-management,* ed. Eugene Pusič. Vol 4. Zagreb, Yugoslavia: Institute for Social Research, University of Zagreb, pp. 177–180.

Aydelotte, M. 1973. *Nursing staffing methodology: a review and critique of selected literature.* Department of Health, Education and Welfare Publication No. NIH 73-433. Washington, D.C.: U.S. Govt. Printing Office.

Bellas, C. 1975. Industrial democracy through worker ownership: an American experience. In *Self-management: economic liberation of man,* ed. J. Vanek. Baltimore: Penguin, pp. 203–212.

Blumberg, P. 1973, *Industrial democracy: the sociology of participation.* New York: Schocken Books.

Braverman, H. 1974. *Labor and monopoly capital: the degradation of work in the twentieth century.* New York: Monthly Review Press.

Bye, B. 1973. *The struggle for workers' participation in Germany.* Chichester, England: Imprint Publications.

Clegg, H. 1960. *A new approach to industrial democracy.* Oxford, England: Basil Blackwell.

Community Health Alternatives Project. 1976. *A search for alternatives to the present health care system.* Washington, D.C.: Institute for Policy Studies.

Denitch, B. 1977. Western Europe's new left socialism. *Working Papers for a New Society* 4: 68–76.

Elvin, R. 1976. Factory power split. *The Guardian* (Manchester, England), January 14.

Employee participation and company structure in the European Community. 1975. *Bulletin of the European Communities.* Supplement (August).

Friedson, E. 1970. *Profession of medicine: a study of the sociology of applied knowledge.* New York: Dodd, Mead.

Garson, J. D. 1972. On the political theory of decentralized socialism. *First international sociological conference on participation and self-management,* ed. Eugene Pusič. Vol. 2. Zagreb, Yugoslavia: Institute for Social Research. University of Zagreb, pp. 82–108.

Garičar, J. 1972. Workers' self-management: ideal type—social reality. *First international sociological conference on participation and self-management,* ed. Eugene Pusič. Vol. 1. Zagreb, Yugoslavia: Institute for Social Research, University of Zagreb, pp. 18–32.

Gorz, A. 1967. *Strategy for labor.* Boston: Beacon Press.

Grand, N. 1976. Nursing ideologies and collective bargaining. In *Management for nurses: a multidisciplinary approach,* ed. S. Stone et al. St. Louis: Mosby, pp. 258–264.

Hays-Bautista, D.; and Harveston, D. Holistic health care. *Social Policy* 7:7–13.

Hillquit, M. 1903. *History of socialism in the United States.* Quoted by H. Laidler in *History of Socialism.* New York: Crowell, 1968.

Jenkins, D. 1973. *Job power.* Baltimore: Penguin.

Jones, F. 1972. Psychiatric treatment centers as therapeutic communities. *First international sociological conference on participation and self-management,* ed. Eugene Pusič. Vol. 4. Zagreb, Yugoslavia: Institute for Social Research, University of Zagreb, pp. 165–176.

Jones, M. 1953. *The therapeutic community.* New York: Basic Books.

Kaplan, B. 1975. Participation and involvement. *Civic Literacy* 1:2.

Kock, S. 1972. Supervision in effective and ineffective hospital wards. *First international sociological conference on participation and self-management,* ed. Eugene Pusič. Vol. 4. Zagreb, Yugoslavia: Institute for Social Research, University of Zagreb, pp. 191–202.

Kolaja, J. 1965. *Workers' councils: the Yugoslav experience.* London: Tavistock Publications.

Mallet, S. 1975. *Essays on the new working class.* St. Louis: Telos Press.

McEwan, J. The cybernetics of self-organizing systems. In *The case for participatory democracy,* ed. G. Benello and D. Roussopoulos. New York: Viking Press.

Mills, C. W. 1953. *White collar.* New York: Oxford Press.

Oakeshott, R. 1975. Mandrago: Spain's oasis of democracy. In *Self-management: economic liberation of man,* ed. J. Vanek. Baltimore: Penguin.

Spiro, M. 1970. *Kibbutz.* New York: Schocken Books.

Supek, R. 1972. Two types of self-managing organizations and technical progress. *First international sociological conference on participation and self-management,* ed. Eugene Pusič. Vol. 2. Zagreb, Yugoslavia: Institute for Social Research, University of Zagreb, pp. 150–173.

Touraine, A. 1966. *Sociologie de l'action.* Paris: Sevil.

Vanek, J. 1975. *Self-management: economic liberation of man.* Baltimore: Penguin.

Veblen, T. 1953. *The theory of the leisure class.* New York: New American Library.

Warner, M. 1974. Whither Yugoslav self-management? Paper presented at the British Sociological Association, February 23, 1974, at London School of Economics, England.

When workers help call the time in management, 1976. *U.S. News and World Report*. May 10.

Whitty, L. 1976. Self-management and the unions in Britain. Paper presented at International Conference on Participatory Democracy in European Firms, July 5, 1976, at Center for Contemporary European Studies, University of Sussex, England.

Zahourek, R. D.; Leone, D.; and Lang, F. 1976. *Creative health services: a model for group nursing practice*. St. Louis: Mosby.

Zaleznik, A. 1976. Power and politics in organizational life. In *Management for nurses: a multidisciplinary approach,* ed. S. Stone et al. St. Louis: Mosby, pp. 13–33.

Chapter 19

Management in Nontraditional Health Care Delivery Systems

Patricia Archbold

OBJECTIVES

After studying this chapter, the learner will:

- Specify three characteristics of a nontraditional health care delivery system
- Identify three special issues confronting managers in nontraditional health care delivery systems
- Describe five steps a manager can take to prevent burnout
- Identify one problem in obtaining community input in planning
- List seven items to note when assessing management in a nontraditional health care delivery system

DEFINITION OF NONTRADITIONAL HEALTH CARE DELIVERY SYSTEM

With the increasing focus on consumerism in health care and the realization that the general well-being of society is directly related to its level of health (Hanlon 1969, p. 96), there has been a dramatic increase in the number of community-based, nontraditional health care delivery systems. A nontraditional health care delivery system is a small system initiated in response to the perceived health care needs of a specific community and outside the aegis of official or traditional voluntary agencies. The new systems range in nature from neighborhood health centers and free clinics to residential treatment centers for addiction problems and daycare centers for the elderly. For the most part they provide primary, restorative, or long-term care to clients from the community. In general, these systems are created to treat an underserved population, facilitate access to health services for a community, and humanize health care delivery to the population served.

Nontraditional health care delivery systems represent attempts to (1) consider the cultural, social, psychological, and physiological aspects of the person; (2) avoid care that is hospital-based and physician-controlled by focusing on wellness in community-based facilities; (3) use health screening, health education, counseling, and referral more deliberately; and (4) utilize social and natural scientists, humanists, health professionals, and consumers in the planning and evaluation of health care (Murray and Zentner 1975, p. 40).

This chapter will focus on several issues in the management of nontraditional health care delivery systems that are unique to these settings: overlapping roles, the "burnout" phenomenon, responsiveness to community needs, and intra- and extra-agency coordination.

OVERLAPPING ROLES

One common characteristic of many nontraditional health care delivery systems is an overlapping of staff functions and a blurring of roles among professional and nonprofessional staff of various academic preparations. Although such overlapping is usually valued by the staff, it can lead to controversy and misunderstanding; when this happens, staff attention and energy must be spent to clarify the issues and roles. For example, the professional staff at a daycare center for adolescents with addiction problems included a pyschologist, social worker, nurse, and three counselors. All of the staff were engaged in counseling and in leading groups. Occasionally the issue of territoriality would be raised when one professional believed his or her domain had been violated by another. This occurred despite the fact that the staff had unanimously agreed that no domain was the property of any one discipline or staff member. The specific issue—who should initiate and lead groups for the families of the clients—created hostility and dissension among the staff until it was brought up at a staff meeting, discussed, and acted upon. A key to successful management in this situation was the provision of a forum for staff discussion of issues.

THE "BURNOUT" PHENOMENON

Another characteristic of nontraditional health care delivery systems is the high level of commitment and dedication of the staff to values that differ from those of the larger society. Staff members often work long hours with less financial reward than they could obtain in a position with a traditional agency. Furthermore, frequent cuts (or threatened cuts) in funding, loss of staff positions, and so forth are an ever present reality for many agencies. Despite the obvious health care needs of the clients, these limitations prevent the delivery of needed services. Recognizing the client problems and wanting to assist in the solutions, yet prevented from taking action because of the lack of funds or personnel, the staff become frustrated. This initial reaction gives way to a feeling of helplessness and a loss of energy known as "burnout." This phenomenon has such physiological manifestations as exhaustion, fatigue, gastrointestinal disturbances, inability to shake a cold, and sleeplessness (Freudenberger 1974, p. 160). This phenomenon occurs with enough regularity so that management tries to take certain preventive measures.

Freudenberger (1974, pp. 162–164) has suggested several methods for preventing burnout, including: (1) training the manager to sift out potentially burned-out persons before they sift themselves out, (2) assisting the training staff to recognize the difference between a realistically and an unrealistically dedicated or committed person, (3) not assigning a staff person to a frustrating task again and again, (4) limiting the number of hours each staff person works, (5) allowing a break or vacation time, (6) maintaining closeness among the staff, (7) encouraging the sharing of experiences among staff members, (8) encouraging the staff to attend workshops and seminars, (9) utilizing more staff or volunteers, and (10) encouraging staff participation in physical exercise. Although these recommendations were made for the volunteer staff of a free clinic, they also apply to both the salaried and volunteer staff of all nontraditional health care delivery systems. Prevention is the best way to deal with burnout.

When a staff person becomes "burned out," the manager should arrange for that person to rest in the form of either a break from the activities that caused the exhaustion or a vacation. Rest and support are necessary to treat this condition.

RESPONSIVENESS TO COMMUNITY NEEDS

Most nontraditional health care delivery systems assume that health care should be arranged to meet the needs and interests of the consumer rather than those of the professional. Consumer input is necessary in order for agencies to respond to community needs. Many problems arise when seeking such input, however. For example, who qualifies as a consumer? The wife of a community physician? The part owner of a local pharmacy? How can one find interested, indigenous community people who will not be intimidated or mystified by the professionals? Not infrequently it is those community groups with special interests that participate in planning. Should these groups be considered as representative of the community served by the facility?

Although these issues are usually the responsibility of the board of directors or administration, managers within nontraditional health agencies take note when the community or staff believe that the needs of the population are not being met. One way to obtain information about this would be to have the clients submit written evaluations of the services.

One can gain useful information if these evaluations are done in conjunction with a statistical survey to determine whether (1) the services are being utilized by a representative group of the population, or (2) whether there are large groups that choose not to use them, or (3) individuals or groups are being excluded from treatment in the facility.

INTRA- AND EXTRAAGENCY COORDINATION

Intraagency functioning in nontraditional health care delivery systems is affected by their size and mission. Because most nontraditional settings are small, with few members, it is possible for many of the staff to participate in the agency's planning process. When this happens, operational goal setting is mutual, and the following benefits result: planning reflects the input of those who will implement it and those who have first-hand knowledge of the problems that might occur in implementation, and the directing function is helped because the implementors have participated in the planning process, thus eliminating any need for the manager to convey the plans to them. One difficulty inherent in this mode of decision making, according to some workers in nontraditional systems, is that the process takes longer when done by a group rather than by an individual. In general, though, it is felt that the advantages outweigh the disadvantages. With this approach the staff needs to be well informed about the issues confronting the system, including its financial status, hiring policies, legal interactions, and so forth.

The staff can become a more cohesive unit during the planning process which is characterized by open discussions. Communication and motivation are two aspects of the directing function that are valued most highly in small, nontraditional health systems; they are engaged in both formally and informally among the staff. The role of director is frequently assumed by different staff members at different times. This flexibility is functional, but reportedly it generates competition among the staff.

The charismatic leader, often a necessary ingredient in the success of a small, nontraditional system, is usually able to hold most of the power in the system. He or she allows "controlled" freedom on the part of the staff. This leader is often a totally dedicated, somewhat controlling person, without whom the agency would have difficulty functioning. He or she usually removes himself or herself from the day-to-day managerial tasks of the organization and concentrates on administrative functions, especially the matter of obtaining funds. In some instances the role of manager may be specifically given to a staff member; however, the managerial tasks are often assumed by the group.

Another aspect of interagency functioning that is characteristic of small, nontraditional agencies is the absence of hierarchy. Whereas the hierarchy of a more traditional agency leads to personal distance, the absence of hierarchy in a nontraditional system fosters personal closeness among the staff. This is further intensified by the social closeness of the staff who take lunch and coffee breaks together, discuss agency business on and off throughout the day, and so forth. This closeness has many advantages, including group support, improved communication among the staff, and the generation of new ideas. It may also create problems. If interpersonal problems arise among the staff, these will affect the day-to-day functioning of the agency. The manager of the agency may also have difficulty discussing the need for improved behavior with a staff member if there is a close friendship between them.

NONTRADITIONAL HEALTH CARE CENTER

To clarify what is meant by nontraditional health care delivery systems, a typical system will be described. There is a small neighborhood health center located in a low-income area of an inner city. Its purpose is to provide humanistic, comprehensive health care to the residents of this community. The idea to create this center came from a public health nurse in the community who rallied support from the members of the community, the city planning commission, and several funding sources. She provided the charismatic leadership to form and maintain the new health center. The system employs seven full-time and four part-time employees, and utilizes the services of ten trained community volunteers as well as a varying number of professional volunteers. The center provides nursing, medical, dental, dietary, pharmacy, and laboratory services. The center is funded through third-party reimbursement and federal and private grants.

The staff of the center believe that certain activities are necessary to meet the goals of the agency, and that any staff member who is qualified may engage in these activities. Consequently, there is a notable overlapping of staff functions within the agency. Generally this overlapping is productive in terms of the center's goals; however, occasionally it becomes necessary for the staff to spend time and energy clarifying certain roles. For example, there was a territorial debate at a staff meeting as to who would make a home visit to a family. The nurse and the social worker both make home visits. In this case, both felt that their expertise was needed to make the assessment, but the agency could not afford to send both on the visit. The issue was resolved at a staff meeting where it was decided that the nurse, who had physical assessment skills, would make the visit after consulting with the social worker about what information she needed. Because these issues are dealt with as they arise in the twice-a-week staff meetings, they do not lead to staff dissension and competition, a possible consequence if not dealt with openly.

The center uses a team approach in the provision of care, which demands a greater emphasis on verbal than on written communication. The absence of hierarchy in this agency has created an intense personal closeness among the staff. They always take coffee and lunch breaks together, and they often discuss work issues among themselves throughout the day. This informal closeness, together with the biweekly staff meetings, is necessary for the team approach to work.

The center staff place a high value on the quality and distribution of health care. Because of their commitment, staff members work long hours with little financial reward. The staff as a whole recognize that preventing burnout is essential for the continued success of the agency. As a group they take steps to make sure that each individual gets enough rest; breaks from difficult, frustrating tasks; and time to attend workshops.

The staff of the center spend more time on activities related to securing and retaining monies and materials than their counterparts in traditional agencies. This occurs in part because there are fewer staff members and so they share these tasks, and in part because the agency depends on outside funding for its survival. One consequence of this dependence is that in order to meet the funding criteria, the agency is drawn into the limitations of the traditional system. There are guidelines, for example, stipulated by state Medicare regulations for administering drugs for certain conditions. The drugs covered by Medicare may not include the drug of choice for the client. Some services that the clinic staff believe are essential are not covered by state and federal insurance programs. Since the staff members have been attracted to the agency because of its avant-garde character, concessions in behavior, treatments, and goals that are made to obtain funding can produce conflict and anger. The management provides a forum to discuss the problems arising from funding concessions and encourages political action to change the funding regulations. Two of the staff members have taken action, through their professional organizations, to obtain third-party payment for needed services.

The center recognizes the importance of consumer input in planning the agency's goals and objectives. The center's advisory board reflects the client population more than most agency boards. The receiving of consumer input is not without problems, however. The barriers in communication that have always existed between the providers of health care and client are found at the center. Mystification by the professionals, even though inadvertent, causes serious problems. The board tries to clarify and validate information exchange. The clarification often takes longer and is more frustrating than other decision-making processes in which professionals and consumers have engaged. Several strategies have been tried to facilitate communication. At first the staff set up orientation programs for the new consumer representatives. When it was realized that this socialization biased the consumer in favor of the value system of the orienters, another approach was tried. The new consumer representatives were given written material on the importance of consumer input and the center's policy of valuing and responding to community needs. Obtaining consumer input is still a problem for the center.

In conclusion, it is apparent that with the diversity of nontraditional health care delivery systems, this brief sketch can give the reader only a very general idea of what is meant by the term. There are many agencies that in no way resemble the neighborhood health center described here.

GUIDELINES FOR ASSESSING MANAGEMENT IN NONTRADITIONAL HEALTH CARE SYSTEMS

The following questions should be answered when assessing management in a nontraditional health care setting:

1 What are the official agency goals?
2 What are the stated goals of the agency according to the staff members?
3 Who participates in setting the goals?
4 What arrangement is made for consumer participation in goal setting?
5 What arrangement is made for staff participation in goal setting?
6 How does managerial decision making occur?
7 Who participates in managerial decision making?
8 How does the system provide for coordination of staff efforts?
9 How are the objectives and task assignments communicated to the staff?
10 What informal means exist for staff coordination?
11 What specific measures are taken to prevent burnout?
12 What evaluation methods are used by the agency?
13 Do the evaluation methods measure goal attainment?

14 Who participates in the evaluation process?
15 How is the evaluation utilized by the agency?

EXERCISES

After assessing the management in a nontraditional health care delivery system of your choice:

1 Observe the behavior of a staff member for an hour. Is it consistent with the goals of the system?
2 Observe a client interacting with the system. Are the interactions consistent with the goals of the agency?
3 Develop two alternative explanations for what you have observed.

SUMMARY

A nontraditional health care delivery system is defined as a small system that has been initiated in response to the perceived health care needs of a specific community and outside the aegis of official or traditional voluntary agencies. The management process within a nontraditional health care system is essentially the same as in other delivery systems. Special issues such as overlapping roles, the burnout phenomenon, intra-agency coordination, and responsiveness to community needs were discussed. An example of a nontraditional health care delivery system was presented in order to elucidate special aspects of management in these systems. Finally, guidelines for the assessment of management within a nontraditional setting were presented and several exercises were suggested.

REFERENCES

Archer, Sarah E.; and Fleshman, Ruth. 1975. Community health nursing: a typology of practice. *Nursing Outlook* 23:358–364.
———. 1976. Community nurse practitioners: another assessment. *Nursing Outlook* 24:499–503.
Arndt, Clara; and Huckabay, Loucine M. Daderian. 1975. *Nursing administration*. St. Louis: Mosby.
Davis, Ann J.; and Underwood, Patricia. 1976. Role, function and decision-making in community mental health. *Nursing Research* 25:256–258.
Freudenberger, Herbert J. 1974. Staff burn-out. *Journal of Social Issues* 30:159–166.
Hanlon, John J. 1969. *Principles of public health administration*. St. Louis: Mosby.

Hitchcock, Janice. 1970. Working in a non-health-oriented setting. *Nursing Clinics of North America* 5,2:251–259.

Leininger, Madeleine. 1973. Open client-centered health care system model. *Nursing Outlook* 23,3:171–173.

Longest, Beaufort. 1976. *Management practices for the health professional.* Reston, Va.: Reston Publishing.

Metsch, Jonathon. 1975. An intersystem perspective for ambulatory care management. *Journal of Nursing Administration* 5,1:33–36.

Murray, Ruth; and Zentner, Judith. 1975. *Nursing concepts for health promotion.* Englewood Cliffs, N.J.: Prentice-Hall.

Chapter 20

Educating Nurses for Leadership

Carolyn Chambers Clark

OBJECTIVES

After studying this chapter, the learner will:

- Define leadership
- List ways in which the teaching-learning process relates to education for leadership
- List several methods that could be used to increase competence in nursing leadership

DEFINITION OF LEADERSHIP

Leadership is a relationship among people that is based upon the willingness of certain people to follow. It is a set of actions on the part of one or more persons that influences members of a group to move toward setting and attaining goals. When leadership is effective, there is goal attainment or output. Leadership implies notions of responsibility, accountability, and power. Accountability means being answerable for one's actions; in nursing it means the collective peer definition of codes of ethics and standards for safe and effective practice. Without accountability, nurses are users, not leaders. Nurse-managers of health care delivery systems and schools of nursing are responsible for accomplishing tasks, as well as for planning and providing growth experiences and rewards or acknowledgment for the group of nurses with which they work. In a similar fashion, nurses in informal leadership positions are responsible for supporting and working with nursing managers and directors rather than complaining about or avoiding work in groups.

Leadership encompasses the wise use of power, managerial functions, and human relations skills (Claus and Bailey 1977, pp. 3–15; Maas and Jacox 1977 pp. 18–19). Nurses exert leadership by helping peers to set meaningful goals; goals serve as the basis for establishing standards. Nurses can exert either informal or formal leadership (as designated leaders) (Clark 1977, p. ix). Nurse-leaders who have formal authority based on their position cannot exert effective leadership without recognizing and supporting the attempts of other nurses who are working to get the job done.

The foundation for personal power is a strong concept of self and growing self-esteem. Nurse-leaders define their own and others' strengths and limitations. They encourage growth in others where limitations are evident and attempt to implement strategies that will enhance strength (Claus and Bailey 1977, pp. 9–10).

Nursing leadership requires knowledge and competence to influence the work environment so that able nurses can realize their potential. Nursing leadership means coordinating others' efforts while remaining committed to organizational goals, and bringing together peer-group efforts to attain goals in a way that no one nurse working alone could accomplish. Nurse-leaders have the skills required to confront subsystems that are fearful of change or that do not know how to grow. Nursing leaders must understand large, complex systems; have the skills required for system intervention; have interpersonal competence in understanding others, providing feedback, disclosing oneself, and managing conflict; have a set of values that has been translated into priorities and action guides with respect to confrontation or support; and have the ability to collect, organize, and transmit information (Bennis 1976, pp. 118–127).

LEADERSHIP AND THE TEACHING-LEARNING PROCESS

Learning is a process that requires change; any process that requires personal change also includes affective components. In nursing, learning is the focus of the struggle to become a functional professional. It is both a vehicle of change and a measure of resistance to change. Learning problems are characteristic, automatic, and inappropriate patterns. They arise from predilections and idiosyncrasies that the teacher and learner bring to the interaction (Ekstein and Wallerstein 1972, pp. 141–158).

Some of the learning problems nurse-educators may identify in students that could interfere with leadership ability are: vigorous denial or skepticism that anything is new or worth learning; attempts to show that the teacher is wrong; dominance or submissiveness; being dependent or trying to have personal needs met to the exclusion of learning; exposing or dwelling upon one's faults; asking to be spoonfed information; having an overinvestment in the course, teacher, or particular method or theory; being underinvolved in or avoiding a course or specific aspect of content; and resisting structure and rules or freedom and choice. Some of the attitudes nurse-educators may bring to the teaching-learning environment that could detract from their teaching are: being the well-intentioned, controlling, all-wise parent; assuming that learning results from the authoritative transmission of technical knowledge and skills; casting the learner in the role of "bad" student; seeing the student as an extension of themselves—as a projection of their power or as proof of their skill as educators; having an overinvestment in certain approaches or theories and not allowing them to be challenged by students; refusing to acknowledge or act upon their own need for continuing education; inducing guilt or using overexplanations when students accuse them of being a disappointment; taking sides with a student against other teachers, or with the administration against students or other teachers.

The model for the teaching-learning process that can prepare nurses for leadership and independent action parallels the model for effective nurse-client interaction. In both cases the helper does not take over the problem, but strengthens others so that they can cope with it themselves. When the nurse-educator responds to student helplessness by attempting to rescue him or her, the student's inherent strength is overlooked. On the other hand, the nurse-educator who provides no structure for learning ignores the student's need for control or structure. Elements of freedom, control, and cognitive-affective-perceptual-motor learning interact with the budding nurse's professional identity as a leader (Clark 1978). The nurse-educator should provide the structure that the student needs. Structured experiences can help the learner master a high level of cognitive complexity, define options within the curriculum, achieve learning goals, reduce anxiety, identify learning problems, match learning styles with learning experiences, and increase contacts with peers. The nurse-educator can encourage students to become self-directed learners and leaders by devising or helping them devise teacher-student learning contracts, by using student input to identify course and learning objectives, by taking risks and modeling leadership strategies, and by accepting the students' divergent ideas. Cognitive-affective-perceptual-motor learning can be enhanced by means of the following experiences: peer teaching and peer supervision; examination of nursing values; problem-centered, mastery learning; and simulated and actual practice in identifying and working through blind spots, learning problems, group and system intervention skills, and conflict management.

Nurse-educators and learners may wish to ask the following questions to determine whether nurses are being educated for leadership:

1   Do nurse-educators "preach" against the director of nursing who clears all decisions through administrators, yet have their own decisions cleared through a nonnurse university administrator?

2   Do nurse-educators assume that a nurse with an advanced degree knows how to teach nurses to be leaders, or is there an ongoing continuing education program for nurse-educators?

3   Do nurse-educators demonstrate competence as group leaders and systems negotiators, or do they have ineffective faculty or faculty-student meetings?

4   Do nursing students learn how to manage by means of practice in simulated and actual situations, or are they taught only theory?

5   Do nursing students learn how to set up and operate their own peer support and review groups, or is the nurse-educator the only one who evaluates practice?

6   Do nurse-educators model how nurse-educator-managers and nursing service managers interface, or do they complain about and blame health care systems or subsystems?

7   Do nurse-educators model personal power by conveying a strong self-concept and predominately high self-esteem, or do they allow others to devalue nursing and nursing actions?

8   Do nurse-educators model manager skills, or do they revert to rescuer or persecutor roles with students?

9   Do nurse-educators introduce change effectively, or do they avoid confrontation?

10   Do nursing students learn how to develop their own reward and praise system, or do competition and negative feedback prevail?

11   Do nursing students learn how to identify and resolve their own learning problems, or are these problems externalized and the blame placed elsewhere?

12   Do some nurse-educators hover over and overcontrol students while others offer no structure for learning, or do the faculty follow consistent, progressive, and planned balance between structure and freedom?

13   Do nurse-educators hint that students should not question their pet theories or interventions, or are divergent thoughts encouraged?

14   Do nurse-educators side with students or administrators, or can they view the system as a whole and act accordingly?

15 Are students told how nurses or nurse-managers "should" act, or does the curriculum include values clarification and values definition in nursing?

16 Are conflicts smoothed over or are they discussed and used as examples of how to manage conflict?

17 Do educators and students view each other as "the enemy," or do both learn how to model empathy and helping skills?

18 Are students required to "read the teacher's mind" and be liked in order to pass a course, or are the course objectives clear and tied to specific learning experiences so that both the students and teacher know what levels of competence need to be reached?

19 Are students told, "You are (will be) a professional, responsible nurse," while being spoonfed theory and overprotected, or are they gradually given increased responsibility and decision-making power as they progress toward graduation?

SUGGESTIONS FOR LEADERSHIP EXPERIENCES

In nursing education it is often assumed that if theories are presented to students and they are told about interventions, they will be able to apply these to a management situation. There is a tendency to undervalue the importance of actual or simulated management experiences. Although some attempts have been made to develop simulated exercises that allow nurses to practice management skills (*You are Barbara Jordan,* 1970), more of these are needed.

More bridges need to be built between theory and practice. One way to do this is to permit students to participate in the academic decision-making process. Students could chair or be more vocal in faculty committee meetings, curriculum meetings, student-faculty meetings, and nurse-educator–nursing service contract meetings. It may be feared that students will take over or be unable to function in more responsible positions, but actually the designated leader is not necessarily the most influential person in a group. Nurse-educators who are competent group leaders and have a strong self-concept can demonstrate leadership skills to students and help them develop their own leadership skills. Deans of nursing schools frequently complain of being overworked and unable to deal with all the system problems they face. One or more students could serve as problem-solvers or form a working committee that would receive problems from the dean and make recommendations or take action to solve these problems. Students could learn more about negotiating systems by being taught how to set up their own clinical or management experiences rather than having the faculty negotiate them with agencies. Students could be helped to offer their theories and knowledge on management to health care agencies in exchange for actual situations in which to practice what they know.

In some states, nursing educators and nursing service personnel are setting up joint demonstration units that have a common philosophy of nursing service, offer a model for delivery, and identify personnel functions and job preparation (Channing, 1976 p. 14). Students could participate actively in this type of planning and thereby gain first-hand knowledge on how to exert nursing leadership.

Argyris's (1977, p. 123) research suggests that the most appropriate learning approach for managers is a double loop one where they invite confrontation, positions are stated so that they can be challenged, and testing is done publicly. Group and intergroup defenses and processes are dealt with as they arise, and games such as camouflaging information are discussed. Argyris's formulations are relevant to nurse-educators and nursing management students. If nurses are to be educated for leadership, they need classroom experiences in double loop learning; nurse-educators might also become better leaders and managers in the process. If students are going to challenge and confront nurse-educators, the latter need to have a strong sense of self and high self-esteem. For nurses to achieve a stronger self-concept, faculty and students may need to investigate valuing processes to determine what they value in nursing. Such a values clarification can be an experience in leadership since it forces nurses to confront their "banal scripts" (Wyckoff 1977, pp. 167–213), which can rob them of their ability to act spontaneously and autonomously on their own behalf. Banal scripts encourage a stilted and repetitive way of acting. In nursing, a banal script would be playing the role of a professional rescuer who works for an institution that is exploitative and pushes workers to their physical limits.

The instructor is not the only one who can evaluate and teach students. Nurse-educators can identify the criterion level of practice in a nursing skill, model it, and then provide structured practice for students until they attain that level. Once a student has achieved skill in that area, he or she can serve as a peer teacher or peer supervisor for one or more other students with minimal direction. This would not only enhance the students' leadership skills, but free the nurse-educator to work with students who need special assistance or to develop new peer teaching or supervisory experiences. Not being able to share leadership, evaluation, and teaching responsibilities with students may indicate a learning problem for nurse-educators who assume that control over evaluation and knowledge is the only way they can exert power and influence. This seems to be a false assumption. Nurse-educators could probably exert even greater influence on nurses' ability to be leaders if they could share influence and leadership.

Nurses also need specific learning experiences in peer review and peer support. Just as they can learn to teach, supervise, and evaluate another nurse's practice, they can learn to work in groups to provide peer review and peer support. However, they need guidelines and a demonstration on how to do this. Toward this end, nurse-educators need to be active and effective participants in their own peer review and peer support groups. Often both students and educators have difficulty giving feedback and criticism. Both may avoid confronting the issue of lack of skill until grading time, or they may be overtly aggressive and attack the other at the time of evaluation.

Students cannot learn how to exert effective leadership in a group of peers unless they have the necessary group skills. Thus, all nurses ought to have specific structured group experiences and preferably a combined theory-clinical course where they could learn group skills and have practice using them. Merely participating in a sensitivity group or taking a course in group dynamics that does not provide structured practice in group leadership will not produce nursing leaders who can work effectively in peer groups.

Likewise, nurses need specific assignments to peer groups. This does not mean telling students to work in groups but then giving them no tools for peer group work. Much of nursing education is competitive. Students compete with one another for grades and teacher approval. Therefore, it is unrealistic to expect that once students graduate, they will be able to work together supportively in health care agencies. The ability to work with others cooperatively and collaboratively does not just appear by magic; it is learned by means of structured learning experiences. If nurse-educators do not have this skill or have not had positive peer group experiences, it will be difficult for them to provide guidelines, rationale, or support for students to develop this skill.

It is expected that nurse practitioners will identify and seek to meet their own learning needs (*Continuing education in nursing,* 1976, p. 6). Yet, not all nursing programs teach students how to do this. This entails learning how to identify learning problems, learning needs, and relevant learning experiences. It requires practice with structured learning experiences and a verbalized rationale as to why these skills are important.

More and more nurse practitioners are establishing private individual or group practices. This calls for specific management skills such as determining the market for a particular service, estimating the initial costs, learning how to obtain a small-business loan, learning the advantages and disadvantages of partnerships and incorporation, and learning how to keep accounts (Simms 1977, p. 114). In addition, the issue of fees and how to determine a reasonable fee structure has to be examined. If nursing students and educators seriously want nurses to become leaders in this area, they ought to develop learning experiences that will prepare nurses to function in private practice.

Even nurses who plan to work in the more traditional health care systems should learn survival strategies and become aware of some of the difficulties they will face. Kramer (1974, 1977) has begun to deal with these issues. Poulin (1977, p. 58) suggests that nurses can develop status and prestige in an organization and prepares the way for them to exert leadership by assuring them that the symbols such as office accouterments and parking space are present, that power centers can be identified, that nurse-managers know how to project the value and significance of nursing, and that they know how to negotiate for an executive title. Gortner (1977, pp. 617–619) lists other survival strategies such as remaining competent, planning the employment interview so that the interviewee asks questions and gets pertinent answers, identifying the fit between the nurse's and the organization's value systems, identifying formal and informal sources of power and authority, being familiar with the principles of organizational innovation and change, deciding what is needed in a system and knowing how to bring about the change, making sure that a problem can be solved, building support systems, and knowing oneself. Calvert (1977, pp. 120–122) points out that women have a particularly difficult time being boss or manager because many people prefer male bosses. Women nurse-managers may need special education on how both women and men prefer (and may coerce) women leaders to be understanding and nurturant. Women nurse-managers will probably need assistance in identifying the internal and external forces that impel them to be nurturant versus their wish to be task-oriented and businesslike. If nurses are to be educated for leadership positions as managers, both educators and students will need to consider and act on their own responsibilities in this area. This closing chapter has tried to draw nurse-educators and nursing students together in the realization that both may need leadership skills. This kind of approach is appropriate for a systems framework where an open system permits a free exchange of resources and information and has the potential for positive feedback leading to change and adaptation.

SUMMARY

Nursing leadership requires knowledge and competence to influence the work environment to enable nurses to reach their full potential. Learning problems can interfere with the process of educating nurses to be leaders. Therefore nurse educators and nursing students must collaborate to identify and decrease these blocks to learning. Simulated and real-life leadership experiences, not just theoretical presentations, ought to be provided for students. Suggestions were made for increasing the number and type of educational leadership experiences for both faculty and students.

REFERENCES

Argyris, Chris. 1977. Double loop learning in organizations. *Harvard Business Review* 55,5:115–125.

Bennis, Warren. 1966. *Beyond bureaucracy: essays on the development and evolution of the human organization.* New York: McGraw-Hill.

———. 1976. New patterns for leadership for tomorrow's organization. In *Management for nurses: a multidisciplinary approach,* ed. Sandra Stone et al. St. Louis: Mosby, pp. 118–127.

Blomgren, George W.; and Thiss, Thomas N. 1976. Awards and incentives can help speed learning. *Training HRD* (December): 28–29.

Calvert, Catherine. 1977. Why a woman can't be a good boss—because no one will let you. *Mademoiselle* (July): 120–122.

Channing, Rose M. 1976. Nursing education and nursing practice in modern partnerships for today and the future. *NJSNA Perspectives* 2,1:9–14.

Clark, Carolyn Chambers. 1977a. Learning to negotiate the system. *Nursing Outlook* 25,1:39–42.

———. 1977b. *The nurse as group leader.* New York: Springer.

———. 1978. *Classroom skills for nurse educators.* New York: Springer.

Claus, Karen E., and Bailey, June T. 1977. *Power and influence in health care: a new approach to leadership.* St. Louis: Mosby.

Continuing education in nursing: guidelines for staff development. 1976. Kansas City, Mo.: American Nurses Association.

Crow, Mary Lynn; and Bonney, Merl E. 1975. Recognizing the authoritarian personality syndrome in educators. *Phi Delta Kappan* (September): 40–44.

DelBueno, Dorothy J. 1976. No more Wednesday matinees! *Nursing Outlook* 24,6:359–361.

DiMarco, N. 1976. Predictors of management training effectiveness for nursing supervisors. *Journal of Continuing Education in Nursing* 7 (July-August):38–46.

Ekstein, Rudolf; and Wallerstein, Robert S. 1972. *The teaching and learning of psychotherapy,* 2nd ed. New York: International Universities Press.

Fiedler, Fred E. 1973. The trouble with leadership training is that it doesn't train leaders. *Psychology Today* (February):23.

Fine, Ruth Barney. 1976. Nursing educators, nursing directors: a symbiotic relationship. *Nurse Educator* 1,3:4–7.

Gall, John. 1977. *Systemantics: how systems work and especially how they fail.* New York: Quadrangle (New York Times).

Gortner, Susan R. 1977. Strategies for survival in the practice world. *American Journal of Nursing* 77,4:618–619.

Grissum, Marlene; and Spengler, Carol. 1976. *Womanpower and health care.* Boston: Little, Brown.

Kohlberg, Lawrence. 1975. The cognitive-developmental approach to moral education. *Phi Delta Kappan* (June):670–678.

Korda, Michael. 1977. The woman who wants to succeed ought to appear in charge. *New York Times* (September 4):1, 10.

Kramer, Marlene. 1974. *Reality shock: why nurses leave nursing.* St. Louis: Mosby.

Kramer, Marlene; and Schmalenberg, Claudia. 1977. The first job: a proving ground, basis for empathy development. *Journal of Nursing Administration* 7,1:13–20.

Maas, Meridean; and Jacox, Ada K. 1977. *Guidelines for nurse autonomy/patient welfare.* New York: Appleton-Century-Crofts.

Poulin, Muriel A. 1977. The nurse administrator: survival in the executive jungle. *Nursing Digest* 5,1:56–58.

Rennels, Max R. 1976. Cerebral symmetry: an urgent concern for education. *Phi Delta Kappan* (March):471–472.

Simmons, Jeanette. 1976. Complex issues facing health education. *American Journal of Public Health* 66,5:429–430.

Simms, Elsie. 1977. Preparation for independent practice. *Nursing Outlook* 25,2:114–118.

Stevens, Barbara. 1975. Management tools needed. *The American Nurse* (April): 9.

You are Barbara Jordan: an in-basket exercise on nursing service administration. 1970. Chicago: Hospital Research and Educational Trust.

Wyckoff, Hogie. 1977. *Solving women's problems.* New York: Grove Press.

Index

When letters are placed with page numbers, the reference is to table *(t.)* or illustration *(i.)*.